UICCInternational Union Against Cancer

TNM
Classification of Malignant Tumours

Edited by

L.H. Sobin, M.K. Gospodarowicz
and
Ch. Wittekind

Seventh Edition
2009

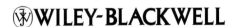

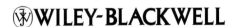WILEY-BLACKWELL

A John Wiley & Sons, Ltd., Publication

This edition first published 2010, © 2010 by Blackwell Publishing Ltd

Blackwell Publishing was acquired by John Wiley & Sons in February 2007. Blackwell's publishing program has been merged with Wiley's global Scientific, Technical and Medical business to form Wiley-Blackwell.

Registered office: John Wiley & Sons Ltd, The Atrium, Southern Gate, Chichester, West Sussex, PO19 8SQ, UK

Editorial offices: 9600 Garsington Road, Oxford, OX4 2DQ, UK
　　　　　　　　　The Atrium, Southern Gate, Chichester, West Sussex, PO19 8SQ, UK
　　　　　　　　　111 River Street, Hoboken, NJ 07030-5774, USA

For details of our global editorial offices, for customer services and for information about how to apply for permission to reuse the copyright material in this book please see our website at www.wiley.com/wiley-blackwell

The right of the author to be identified as the author of this work has been asserted in accordance with the Copyright, Designs and Patents Act 1988.

Library of Congress Cataloging-in-Publication Data

TNM classification of malignant tumours / edited by L.H. Sobin, M.K. Gospodarowicz, and Ch. Wittekind. — 7th ed.
　　p. ; cm.
　At head of title: UICC International Union Against Cancer.
　Includes bibliographical references.
　ISBN 978-1-4443-3241-4
1. Tumors—Classification.　I. Sobin, L. H.　II. Gospodarowicz, M. K. (Mary K.)　III. Wittekind, Ch. (Christian)　IV. International Union against Cancer.　V. Title: Classification of malignant tumours.
　[DNLM: 1. Neoplasms—classification. QZ 15 T626 2009]
　RC258.T583 2009
　616.99'40012—dc22

　　　　　　　　　　　　　　　　　　　　　　　　　　　　　　　　　　　　　2009029889

A catalogue record for this book is available from the British Library.

Set in Frutiger 9.5/12 pt by Macmillan Publishing Solutions

Printed & bound in Spain

2　2010

*They are called wise
who put things in their right order*
—*Thomas Aquinas*

EDITORS

L.H. Sobin, M.D.
Division of Gastrointestinal Pathology
Armed Forces Institute of Pathology
Washington, D.C. 20306, USA

M.K. Gospodarowicz, M.D.
Department of Radiation Oncology
University of Toronto,
Princess Margaret Hospital
Toronto, Canada

Prof. Dr. med. Ch. Wittekind
Institut für Pathologie des
Universitätsklinikums Leipzig
Liebigstraße 26
D-04103 Leipzig, Germany

CONTENTS

PREFACE

In the seventh edition of the *TNM Classification* many of the tumour sites have remained unchanged from the sixth edition.[1] However, some tumour entities and anatomic sites have been newly introduced and some tumours contain modifications: this follows the basic philosophy of maintaining stability of the classification over time. The modifications and additions reflect new data on prognosis, as well as new methods for assessing prognosis.[2] Some changes have already appeared in the *TNM Supplement*[3] as proposals. Subsequent support warrants their incorporation into the classification.

The major alterations concern carcinomas of the oesophagus and the oesophagogastric junction, stomach, lung, appendix, biliary tract, skin carcinoma, and prostate. There are several new classifications: gastrointestinal carcinoids (neuroendocrine tumours), gastrointestinal stromal tumour, upper aerodigestive mucosal melanoma, Merkel cell carcinoma, uterine sarcomas, intrahepatic cholangiocarcinoma, and adrenal cortical carcinoma.

A new approach has been adopted to separate stage groupings from prognostic groupings in which other prognostic factors are added to T, N, and M categories. These new prognostic groupings are presented for oesophagus and prostate.

Except for the presentation of both stage groupings and prognostic groupings at the sites mentioned above, the International Union Against Cancer (UICC)

TNM Classification is identical to that published by the American Joint Committee on Cancer (AJCC).[4] This is the result of the intent to have only one standard and reflects the collaborative efforts made by all national TNM committees to achieve uniformity in this field.

Changes made between the sixth and seventh editions are indicated by a bar at the left-hand side of the text. To avoid ambiguity, users are encouraged to cite the year of the TNM publication they have used in their list of references.

A TNM homepage on the Internet with Frequently Asked Questions (FAQs) and a form for submitting questions or comments on the TNM can be found at: http://www.uicc.org.

The UICC's TNM Prognostic Factors Project has instituted a process for evaluating proposals to improve the *TNM Classification*. This procedure aims at a continuous systematic approach composed of two arms: (1) procedures to address formal proposals from investigators, and (2) a periodic literature search for articles concerning improvements to TNM. The proposals and results of the literature search are evaluated by members of a UICC panel of experts as well as by the TNM Prognostic Factors Project Committee members. The national TNM Committees including the American Joint Committee on Cancer participated in this process. More details and a checklist that will facilitate the formulation of proposals can be obtained at http://www. uicc.org.

International Union Against Cancer (UICC)
62, route de Frontenex
CH-1207 Geneva, Switzerland
Fax ++41 22 8091810

[1] International Union Against Cancer (UICC). *TNM Classification of Malignant Tumours*, 6th ed. Sobin LH, Wittekind Ch., eds. New York: Wiley; 2002.

[2] International Union Against Cancer (UICC). *Prognostic Factors in Cancer*, 3rd ed. Gospodarowicz MK, O'Sullivan B, Sobin LH, eds. New York: Wiley; 2006.

[3] International Union Against Cancer (UICC). *TNM Supplement. A Commentary on Uniform Use*, 3rd ed. Wittekind Ch, Henson DE, Hutter RVP, et al., eds. New York; Wiley; 2003.

[4] American Joint Committee on Cancer (AJCC). *Cancer Staging Manual* 7th ed. Edge SB, Byrd DR, Carducci MA, Compton CC, Fritz AG, Greene F, Trotti A. eds. New York: Springer; 2009.

ACKNOWLEDGEMENTS

The Editors have much pleasure in acknowledging the great help received from the members of the TNM Prognostic Factors Project Committee and the National Staging Committees Global Representatives and international organizations listed on pages xvii–xix.

Professor Paul Hermanek has continued to provide encouragement and valuable criticism.

The seventh edition of the *TNM Classification* is the result of a number of consultative meetings organized and supported by the UICC and AJCC secretariats.

This publication was made possible by grants 1U58DP001819-01, HR/CCH 013713 and HR3/CCH417470 from the Centers for Disease Control and Prevention (CDC) (USA). Its contents are solely the responsibility of the authors and do not necessarily represent the official views of the CDC.

ABBREVIATIONS

a	autopsy, p. 17
c	clinical, p. 8, 10
C	certainty factor, p. 17–18
G	histopathological grading, p. 16
ICD-O	*International Classification of Diseases for Oncology*, 3rd ed., 2000
ITC	isolated tumour cells, p. 13–14
L	lymphatic invasion, p. 17
m	multiple tumours, p. 9
M	distant metastasis
N	regional lymph node metastasis
p	pathological, p. 12
Pn	perineural invasion, p. 17
r	recurrent tumour, p. 17
R	residual tumour after treatment, p. 18–19
sn	sentinel lymph node, p. 13
Stage	anatomical Stage, p. 19
T	extent of primary tumour
V	venous invasion, p. 17
y	classification after initial multimodality treatment, p. 16

ORGANIZATIONS ASSOCIATED WITH THE TNM SYSTEM

CDC   Centers for Disease Control and Prevention (USA)

FIGO   International Federation of Gynaecology and Obstetrics

IASLC   International Association for the Study of Lung Cancer

WHO   World Heath Organization

National Committees

Australia and New Zealand:	National TNM Committee
Austria, Germany, Switzerland:	Deutschsprachiges TNM-Komitee
Belgium:	National TNM Committee
Brazil:	National TNM Committee
Canada:	National Staging Advisory Committee
India:	National TNM Committee
Italy:	Italian Prognostic Systems Project
Japan:	Japanese Joint Committee
Latin America and Caribbean:	Sociedad Latinoamericana y del Caribe de Oncología Médica
Poland:	National Staging Committee
Singapore:	National Staging Committee

Spain:	National Staging Committee
South Africa:	National Staging Committee
United Kingdom:	National Staging Committee
United States of America:	American Joint Committee on Cancer

MEMBERS OF UICC COMMITTEES ASSOCIATED WITH THE TNM SYSTEM

In 1950 the UICC appointed a Committee on Tumour Nomenclature and Statistics. In 1954 this Committee became known as the Committee on Clinical Stage Classification and Applied Statistics and in 1966 it was named the Committee on TNM Classification. Taking into consideration new factors of prognosis the Committee was named in 1994 the TNM Prognostic Factors Project Committee, and in 2003 the main committee was named 'TNM Prognostic Factors Core Group'.

UICC TNM Prognostic Factors Core Group: 2009

Asamura, H.	Japan
Brierley, J.	Canada
Denis, L.	Belgium
Gospodarowicz, M.K.	Canada
Greene, F.L.	USA
Groome, P.	Canada
Mason, M.	UK
O'Sullivan, B.	Canada
Odicino, F.	Italy
Sobin, L.H.	USA
Wittekind, Ch.	Germany

Previous members

Anderson, W.A.D.	USA
Baclesse, F.	France
Badellino, F.	Italy
Barajas-Vallejo, E.	Mexico
Benedet, J.L.	Canada
Benhamou-Borowski, E.	France
Blinov, N.	Russia
Bucalossi, P.	Italy
Burn, I.	United Kingdom
Bush, R.S.	Canada
Carr, D.T.	USA
Copeland, M.M.	USA
Costachel, O.	Romania
Delafresnaye, J.	France
Denoix, P.	France
Fischer, A.W.	Federal Republic of Germany
Fleming, I.D.	USA
Gentil, F.	Brazil
Ginsberg, R.	Canada
Hamperl, H.	Federal Republic of Germany
Harmer, M.H.	United Kingdom
Hayat, M.	France
Henson, D.E.	USA
Hermanek, P.	Germany
Hultberg, S.	Sweden
Hutter, R.V.P.	USA
Ichikawa, H.	Japan
Imai, T.	Japan
Ishikawa, S.	Japan
Junqueira, A.C.C.	Brazil
Kasdorf, H.	Uruguay
Kottmeier, H.L.	Sweden
Koszarowski, T.	Poland

SECTION EDITORS

General Rules	L. H. Sobin, J. Brierley, M.K. Gospodarowicz, B. O'Sullivan
Head and Neck	B. O'Sullivan
Thyroid	J. Brierley
Upper Gastrointestinal Tract	Ch. Wittekind, S. Yamasaki
Lower Gastrointestinal Tract	L.H. Sobin, J. Brierley
Lung	P. Goldstraw, P. Groome
Bone and Soft Tissues	B. O'Sullivan
Skin	F.L. Greene
Breast	F.L. Greene
Gynaecological Tumours	F. Odicino
Genitourinary Tumours	M.K. Gospodarowicz
Ophthalmic Tumours	Ch. Wittekind
Malignant Lymphoma	M.K. Gospodarowicz

UICC TNM expert panel members,
see http://www.uicc.org

INTRODUCTION

The History of the TNM System

The TNM System for the classification of malignant tumours was developed by Pierre Denoix (France) between the years 1943 and 1952.[1]

In 1950, the UICC appointed a Committee on Tumour Nomenclature and Statistics and adopted, as a basis for its work on clinical stage classification, the general definitions of local extension of malignant tumours suggested by the World Health Organization (WHO) Sub-Committee on The Registration of Cases of Cancer as well as Their Statistical Presentation.[2]

In 1953, the Committee held a joint meeting with the International Commission on Stage-Grouping in Cancer and Presentation of the Results of Treatment of Cancer appointed by the International Congress of Radiology. Agreement was reached on a general technique for classification by anatomical extent of the disease, using the TNM system.

In 1954, the Research Commission of the UICC set up a special Committee on Clinical Stage Classification and Applied Statistics to 'pursue studies in this field

---

[1] Denoix PF. Nomenclature des cancers. *Bull Inst Nat Hyg (Paris)* 1944:69–73; 1945:82–84; 1950:81–84; 1952:743–748.
[2] World Health Organization. Technical Report Series, Number 53, July 1952, pp. 47–48.

and to extend the general technique of classification to cancer at all sites'.

In 1958, the Committee published the first recommendations for the clinical stage classification of cancers of the breast and larynx and for the presentation of results.[3]

A second publication in 1959 presented revised proposals for the breast, for clinical use and evaluation over a 5-year period (1960–1964).[4]

Between 1960 and 1967, the Committee published nine brochures describing proposals for the classification of 23 sites. It was recommended that the classification proposals for each site be subjected to prospective or retrospective trial for a 5-year period.

In 1968, these brochures were combined in a booklet, the *Livre de Poche*[5] and a year later, a complementary booklet was published detailing recommendations for the setting-up of field trials, for the presentation of end results and for the determination and expression of cancer survival rates.[6] The *Livre de Poche* was subsequently translated into 11 languages.

---

[3] International Union Against Cancer (UICC). Committee on Clinical Stage Classification and Applied Statistics. *Clinical Stage Classification and Presentation of Results, Malignant Tumours of the Breast and Larynx*. Paris; 1958.

[4] International Union Against Cancer (UICC). Committee on Stage Classification and Applied Statistics. *Clinical Stage Classification and Presentation of Results, Malignant Tumours of the Breast*. Paris; 1959.

[5] International Union Against Cancer (UICC). *TNM Classification of Malignant Tumours*. Geneva; 1968.

[6] International Union Against Cancer (UICC). *TNM General Rules*. Geneva; 1969

In 1974 and 1978, second and third editions[7,8] were published containing new site classifications and amendments to previously published classifications. The third edition was enlarged and revised in 1982. It contained new classifications for selected tumours of childhood. This was carried out in collaboration with La Societe Internationale d'Oncologie Pediatrique (SIOP). A classification of ophthalmic tumours was published separately in 1985.

Over the years some users introduced variations in the rules of classification of certain sites. In order to correct this development, the antithesis of standardization, the national TNM committees in 1982 agreed to formulate a single TNM. A series of meetings was held to unify and update existing classifications as well as to develop new ones. The result was the fourth edition of TNM.[9]

In 1993, the project published the *TNM Supplement*.[10] The purpose of this work was to promote the uniform use of TNM by providing detailed explanations of the TNM rules with practical examples. It also included proposals for new classifications and

[7] International Union Against Cancer (UICC). *TNM Classification of Malignant Tumours*, 2nd ed. Geneva; 1974.

[8] International Union Against Cancer (UICC): *TNM Classification of Malignant Tumours*, 3rd ed. Harmer MH, ed. Geneva; 1978. Enlarged and revised 1982.

[9] International Union Against Cancer (UICC). *TNM Classification of Malignant Tumours*, 4th ed. Hermanek P, Sobin LH, eds. Heidelberg: Springer; 1987. Revised 1992.

[10] International Union Against Cancer (UICC). *TNM Supplement. A Commentary on Uniform Use*. Hermanek P, Henson DE, Hutter RVP, et al., eds. Heidelberg: Springer; 1993.

optional expansions of selected categories. Second and third editions appeared in 2001[11] and 2003.[12]

In 1995, the project published *Prognostic Factors in Cancer*,[13] a compilation and discussion of prognostic factors in cancer, both anatomic and non-anatomic, at each of the body sites. This was expanded in the second edition in 2001[14] with emphasis on the relevance of different prognostic factors. The subsequent third edition in 2006[15] attempted to refine this by providing evidence-based criteria for relevance.

The present seventh edition of *TNM Classification* contains rules of classification and staging that correspond with those appearing in the seventh edition of the *AJCC Cancer Staging Manual* (2009)[16] and have approval of all national TNM committees. These are listed on pages. xv–xvi., together with the names of members of the UICC committees who have been associated with the TNM system. The UICC recognizes the need for stability

[11] International Union Against Cancer (UICC). *TNM Supplement. A Commentary on Uniform Use*, 2nd ed. Wittekind Ch, Henson DE, Hutter RVP, et al., eds. New York: Wiley; 2001.

[12] International Union Against Cancer (UICC). *TNM Supplement. A Commentary on Uniform Use*, 3rd ed. Wittekind Ch, Green FL, Henson DE, et al., eds. New York: Wiley; 2003.

[13] International Union Against Cancer (UICC). *Prognostic Factors in Cancer*. Hermanek P, Gospodarowicz MK, Henson DE, et al., eds. Berlin, Heidelberg, New York: Springer; 1995.

[14] International Union Against Cancer (UICC). Prognostic Factors in Cancer, 2nd ed. Gospodarowicz MK, Henson DE, Hutter RVP, et al., eds. New York: Wiley; 2001.

[15] International Union Against Cancer (UICC). *Prognostic Factors in Cancer*, 3rd ed. Gospodarowicz MK, O'Sullivan B, Sobin LH, eds. New York: Wiley; 2006.

[16] American Joint Committee on Cancer (AJCC). *AJCC Cancer Staging Manual*, 7th ed. Edge SB, Byrd DR, Carducci MA, et al., eds. New York: Springer; 2009.

in the TNM classification so that data can be accumulated in an orderly way over reasonable periods of time. Accordingly, it is the intention that the classifications published in this booklet should remain unchanged until some major advances in diagnosis or treatment relevant to a particular site requires reconsideration of the current classification.

To develop and sustain a classification system acceptable to all requires the closest liaison between national and international committees. Only in this way will all oncologists be able to use a 'common language' in comparing their clinical material and in assessing the results of treatment. While the classification is based on published evidence, in areas of controversy it is based on international consensus.

The continuing objective of the UICC is to achieve common consent in the classification of anatomical extent of disease.

The Principles of the TNM System

The practice of dividing cancer cases into groups according to so-called stages arose from the fact that survival rates were higher for cases in which the disease was localized than for those in which the disease had extended beyond the organ of origin. These groups were often referred to as early cases and late cases, implying some regular progression with time. Actually, the stage of disease at the time of diagnosis may be a reflection not only of the rate of growth and extension of the neoplasm but also of the type of tumour and of the tumour–host relationship.

The anatomical staging of cancer is hallowed by tradition, and for the purpose of analysis of groups of patients it is often necessary to use such a method. The UICC believes that it is important to reach agreement on the recording of accurate information on the anatomical extent of the disease for each site, because the precise clinical description of malignant neoplasms and histopathological classification may serve a number of related objectives, namely:

1. To aid the clinician in the planning of treatment
2. To give some indication of prognosis
3. To assist in evaluation of the results of treatment
4. To facilitate the exchange of information between treatment centres
5. To contribute to the continuing investigation of human cancer
6. To support cancer control activities

The principal purpose to be served by international agreement on the classification of cancer cases by extent of disease is to provide a method of conveying clinical experience to others without ambiguity.

There are many bases or axes of tumour classification, e.g., the anatomical site and the clinical and pathological extent of disease, the reported duration of symptoms or signs, the gender and age of the patient, and the histological type and grade. All of these bases or axes represent variables that are known to have an influence on the outcome of the disease. Classification by anatomical extent of disease as determined clinically and histopathologically is the one with which the TNM system primarily deals.

The clinician's immediate task is to make a judgement as to prognosis and a decision as to the most effective course of treatment. This judgement and this decision require, among other things, an objective assessment of the anatomical extent of the disease. In accomplishing this, the trend is away from 'staging' to meaningful description, with or without some form of summarization.

To meet the stated objectives a system of classification is needed:

1. whose basic principles are applicable to all sites regardless of treatment; and
2. which may be supplemented later by information that becomes available from histopathology and/or surgery.

The TNM system meets these requirements.

> *Substantial changes in the 2009 seventh edition compared to the 2002 sixth edition are marked by a bar at the left-hand side of the page.*

The General Rules of the TNM System

The TNM system for describing the anatomical extent of disease is based on the assessment of three components:

T – The extent of the primary tumour
N – The absence or presence and extent of regional lymph node metastasis
M – The absence or presence of distant metastasis

The addition of numbers to these three components indicates the extent of the malignant disease, thus:

    T0, T1, T2, T3, T4   N0, N1, N2, N3   M0, M1

In effect the system is a 'shorthand notation' for describing the extent of a particular malignant tumour.

The general rules applicable to all sites are as follows:

1. All cases should be confirmed microscopically. Any cases not so proved must be reported separately.
2. Two classifications are described for each site, namely:

    (a) Clinical classification: the pretreatment clinical classification) designated TNM (or cTNM) is essential to select and evaluate therapy. This is based on evidence acquired before treatment. Such evidence arises from physical examination, imaging, endoscopy, biopsy, surgical exploration, and other relevant examinations.

    (b) Pathological classification: the postsurgical histopathological classification, designated pTNM, is used to guide adjuvant therapy and provides additional data to estimate prognosis and calculate end results. This is based on evidence acquired before treatment, supplemented or modified by additional evidence acquired from surgery and from pathological examination. The pathological assessment of the primary tumour (pT) entails a resection of the primary tumour or biopsy adequate to evaluate the highest pT category. The pathological assessment of the regional lymph nodes (pN) entails removal of the lymph nodes adequate to validate the absence of regional lymph node metastasis (pN0) or sufficient to evaluate the highest pN category. An excisional biopsy of a lymph node without pathological assessment of the primary is insufficient to fully evaluate the pN category

and is a clinical classification. The pathological assessment of distant metastasis (pM) entails microscopic examination.

3. After assigning T, N, and M and/or pT, pN, and pM categories, these may be grouped into stages. The TNM classification and stage groups, once established, must remain unchanged in the medical records.

Clinical and pathological data may be combined when only partial information is available either in the pathological classification or the clinical classification.

4. If there is doubt concerning the correct T, N, or M category to which a particular case should be allotted, then the lower (i.e., less advanced) category should be chosen. This will also be reflected in the stage grouping.

5. In the case of multiple primary tumours in one organ, the tumour with the highest T category should be classified and the multiplicity or the number of tumours should be indicated in parenthesis, e.g., T2(m) or T2(5). In simultaneous bilateral primary cancers of paired organs, each tumour should be classified independently. In tumours of the liver, ovary, and fallopian tube, multiplicity is a criterion of T classification, and in tumours of the lung multiplicity may be a criterion of T or M classification.

6. Definitions of TNM categories and stage grouping may be telescoped or expanded for clinical or research purposes as long as the basic definitions recommended are not changed. For instance, any T, N, or M can be divided into subgroups.

For more details on classification the reader is referred to the *TNM Supplement*.

Anatomical Regions and Sites

The sites in this classification are listed by code number of the International Classification of Diseases for Oncology.[17] Each region or site is described under the following headings:

- Rules for classification with the procedures for assessing the T, N, and M categories
- Anatomical sites, and subsites if appropriate
- Definition of the regional lymph nodes
- TNM Clinical classification
- pTNM Pathological classification
- G Histopathological grading
- Stage grouping
- Summary

TNM Clinical Classification

The following general definitions are used throughout:

T – Primary Tumour

TX   Primary tumour cannot be assessed
T0   No evidence of primary tumour
Tis   Carcinoma in situ

T1–T4 Increasing size and/or local extent of the primary tumour

---

[17] *WHO International Classification of Diseases for Oncology ICD-O*, 3rd ed. Fritz A, Percy C, Jack A, et al., eds. Geneva: WHO; 2000.

N – Regional Lymph Nodes

NX   Regional lymph nodes cannot be assessed
N0   No regional lymph node metastasis
N1–N3 Increasing involvement of regional lymph nodes

M – Distant Metastasis*

M0   No distant metastasis
M1   Distant metastasis

Note: *The MX category is considered to be inappropriate as clinical assessment of metastasis can be based on physical examination alone. (The use of MX may result in exclusion from staging.)

The category M1 may be further specified according to the following notation:

Pulmonary	PUL (C34)	Bone marrow	MAR (C42.1)
Osseous	OSS (C40, 41)	Pleura	PLE (C38.4)
Hepatic	HEP (C22)	Peritoneum	PER (C48.1,2)
Brain	BRA (C71)	Adrenals	ADR (C74)
Lymph nodes	LYM (C77)	Skin	SKI (C44)
Others	OTH		

Subdivisions of TNM

Subdivisions of some main categories are available for those who need greater specificity (e.g., T1a, T1b, or N2a, N2b).

pTNM Pathological Classification

The following general definitions are used throughout:

pT – Primary Tumour

pTX   Primary tumour cannot be assessed histologically

pT0   No histological evidence of primary tumour

pTis   Carcinoma in situ

pT1–4   Increasing size and/or local extent of the primary tumour histologically

pN – Regional Lymph Nodes

pNX   Regional lymph nodes cannot be assessed histologically

pN0   No regional lymph node metastasis histologically

pN1–3   Increasing involvement of regional lymph nodes histologically

Notes: 1. Direct extension of the primary tumour into lymph nodes is classified as lymph node metastasis.

2. Tumour deposits (satellites), i.e., macro- or microscopic nests or nodules, in the lymph drainage area of a primary carcinoma without histological evidence of residual lymph node in the nodule, may represent discontinuous spread, venous invasion (V1/2) or a totally replaced lymph node. If a nodule is considered by the pathologist to be a totally replaced lymph node (generally having a smooth contour), it should be recorded as a positive lymph node, and each such nodule should be counted separately as a lymph node in the final pN determination.

3. Metastasis in any lymph node other than regional is classified as a distant metastasis.
4. When size is a criterion for pN classification, measurement is made of the metastasis, not of the entire lymph node.
5. Cases with micrometastasis only, i.e., no metastasis larger than 0.2 cm, can be identified by the addition of ' (mi)', e.g., pN1(mi).
6. The number of resected and positive nodes should be recorded.

Sentinel Lymph Node

The sentinel lymph node is the first lymph node to receive lymphatic drainage from a primary tumour. If it contains metastatic tumour this indicates that other lymph nodes may contain tumour. If it does not contain metastatic tumour, other lymph nodes are not likely to contain tumour. Occasionally there is more than one sentinel lymph node.

The following designations are applicable when sentinel lymph node assessment is attempted:

pNX(sn)   Sentinel lymph node could not be assessed
pN0(sn)   No sentinel lymph node metastasis
pN1(sn)   Sentinel lymph node metastasis

Isolated Tumour Cells

Isolated tumour cells (ITC) are single tumour cells or small clusters of cells not more than 0.2 mm in greatest extent that can be detected by routine H and E stains or immunohistochemistry. An additional criterion has been proposed to include a cluster of fewer than 200 cells in a single histological cross-section. ITCs do not typically show evidence of metastatic activity (e.g., proliferation or stromal reaction) or penetration of vascular or lymphatic sinus walls. Cases with ITC in lymph nodes or at distant sites should be classified as N0 or M0, respectively. The same applies to cases with findings suggestive of tumour cells or their components by non-morphological techniques such as flow cytometry or DNA analysis. These cases should be analysed separately.[18] Their classification is as follows:

pN0	No regional lymph node metastasis histologically, no examination for isolated tumour cells (ITC)
pN0(i−)	No regional lymph node metastasis histologically, negative morphological findings for ITC
pN0(i+)	No regional lymph node metastasis histologically, positive morphological findings for ITC
pN0(mol−)	No regional lymph node metastasis histologically, negative non-morphological findings for ITC
pN0(mol+)	No regional lymph node metastasis histologically, positive non-morphological findings for ITC

[18] Hermanek P, Hutter RVP, Sobin LH, Wittekind Ch. Classification of isolated tumour cells and micrometastasis. *Cancer* 1999; 86:2668–2673

Cases with or examined for isolated tumour cells in sentinel lymph nodes can be classified as follows:

pN0(i–)(sn) No sentinel lymph node metastasis histologically, negative morphological findings for ITC

pN0(i+)(sn) No sentinel lymph node metastasis histologically, positive morphological findings for ITC

pN0(mol–)(sn) No sentinel lymph node metastasis histologically, negative non-morphological findings for ITC

pN0(mol+)(sn) No sentinel lymph node metastasis histologically, positive non-morphological findings for ITC

pM – Distant Metastasis*

pM1 Distant metastasis microscopically confirmed

Note: *pM0 and pMX are not valid categories.

The category pM1 may be further specified in the same way as M1 (see page 11).

Isolated tumour cells found in bone marrow with morphological techniques are classified according to the scheme for N, e.g., M0(i+). For non-morphologic findings 'mol' is used in addition to M0, e.g., M0(mol+).

Histopathological Grading

In most sites further information regarding the primary tumour may be recorded under the following heading:

G – Histopathological Grading

GX	Grade of differentiation cannot be assessed
G1	Well differentiated
G2	Moderately differentiated
G3	Poorly differentiated
G4	Undifferentiated

Notes: Grades 3 and 4 can be combined in some circumstances as 'G3–4, poorly differentiated or undifferentiated.'
The bone and soft tissue sarcoma classifications also use 'high grade' and 'low grade'.
Special systems of grading are recommended for tumours of breast, corpus uteri, prostate, and liver.

Additional Descriptors

For identification of special cases in the TNM or pTNM classification, the m, y, r, and a symbols may be used. Although they do not affect the stage grouping, they indicate cases needing separate analysis.

m Symbol. The suffix m, in parentheses, is used to indicate the presence of multiple primary tumours at a single site. See TNM rule no. 5. (See page 9)

y Symbol. In those cases in which classification is performed during or following multimodality therapy, the cTNM or pTNM category is identified by a y prefix. The ycTNM or ypTNM categorizes the extent of tumour actually present at the time of that examination.

The y categorization is not an estimate of the extent of tumour prior to multimodality therapy.

r Symbol. Recurrent tumours, when classified after a disease-free interval, are identified by the prefix r.

a Symbol. The prefix a indicates that classification is first determined at autopsy.

Optional Descriptors

L – Lymphatic Invasion

LX   Lymphatic invasion cannot be assessed
L0   No lymphatic invasion
L1   Lymphatic invasion

V – Venous Invasion

VX   Venous invasion cannot be assessed
V0   No venous invasion
V1   Microscopic venous invasion
V2   Macroscopic venous invasion

Note: Macroscopic involvement of the wall of veins (with no tumour within the veins) is classified as V2.

Pn – Perineural Invasion

PnX   Perineural invasion cannot be assessed
Pn0   No perineural invasion
Pn1   Perineural invasion

C-Factor

The C-factor, or certainty factor, reflects the validity of classification according to the diagnostic methods employed. Its use is optional.

The C-factor definitions are:

C1   Evidence from standard diagnostic means (e.g., inspection, palpation, and standard radiography, intraluminal endoscopy for tumours of certain organs)

C2   Evidence obtained by special diagnostic means (e.g., radiographic imaging in special projections, tomography, computerized tomography [CT], ultrasonography, lymphography, angiography; scintigraphy; magnetic resonance imaging [MRI]; endoscopy, biopsy, and cytology)

C3   Evidence from surgical exploration, including biopsy and cytology

C4   Evidence of the extent of disease following definitive surgery and pathological examination of the resected specimen

C5   Evidence from autopsy

Example: Degrees of C may be applied to the T, N, and M categories. A case might be described as T3C2, N2C1, M0C2.

The TNM clinical classification is therefore equivalent to C1, C2, and C3 in varying degrees of certainty, while the pTNM pathological classification generally is equivalent to C4.

Residual Tumour (R) Classification*

The absence or presence of residual tumour after treatment is described by the symbol R. More details can be found in the *TNM Supplement* (see Preface, footnote 3).

TNM and pTNM describe the anatomical extent of cancer in general without considering treatment. They can be supplemented by the R classification, which deals with tumour status after treatment. It reflects the effects of therapy, influences further therapeutic procedures and is a strong predictor of prognosis.

The definitions of the R categories are:

RX   Presence of residual tumour cannot be assessed
R0   No residual tumour
R1   Microscopic residual tumour
R2   Macroscopic residual tumour

Note: *Some consider the R classification to apply only to the primary tumour and its local or regional extent. Others have applied it more broadly to include distant metastasis. The specific usage should be indicated when the R is used.

Stage Grouping

The TNM system is used to describe and record the anatomical extent of disease. For purposes of tabulation and analysis it is useful to condense these categories into stage groups. For consistency, in the TNM system, carcinoma in situ is categorized Stage 0; in general, tumours localized to the organ of origin as Stages I and II, locally extensive spread, particularly to regional lymph nodes as Stage III, and those with distant metastasis as Stage IV. The stage adopted is such as to ensure, as far as possible, that each group is more or less homogeneous in respect of survival, and that the survival rates of these groups for each cancer site are distinctive.

For pathological stage groups, if sufficient tissue has been removed for pathological examination to evaluate the highest T and N categories, M1 may be either clinical (cM1) or pathological (pM1). However, if only a distant metastasis has had microscopic confirmation, the classification is pathological (pM1) and the stage is pathological.

Although the anatomical extent of disease, as categorized by TNM, is a very powerful prognostic indicator in cancer, it is recognized that many factors have a significant impact on predicting outcomes. Some have been incorporated into stage grouping, as has grade in soft tissue sarcoma and age in thyroid cancer. These classifications will be unchanged in this edition. In the newly revised classifications for oesophagus and prostate carcinomas, *stage grouping* has been maintained as defining the anatomical extent of disease and new *prognostic groupings* that incorporate other prognostic factors have been proposed.

Site Summary

As an aide-memoir or as a means of reference, a simple summary of the chief points that distinguish the most important categories is added at the end of each site. These abridged definitions are not completely adequate, and the full definitions should always be consulted.

Related Classifications

Since 1958, WHO has been involved in a programme aimed at providing internationally acceptable criteria for the histological diagnosis of tumours. This has resulted in the *International Histological Classification of Tumours*, which contains, in an illustrated multivolume series, definitions of tumour types and a proposed nomenclature. A new series, *WHO Classification of Tumours—Pathology and Genetics of Tumours*, continues this effort. (Information on these publications is at http://www.iarc.fr.)

The *WHO International Classification of Diseases for Oncology (ICD-O)* (see footnote, page 10) is a coding system for neoplasms by topography and morphology and for indicating behaviour (e.g., malignant, benign). This coded nomenclature is identical in the morphology field for neoplasms to the *Systematized Nomenclature of Medicine* (SNOMED).[19]

In the interest of promoting national and international collaboration in cancer research and specifically of facilitating cooperation in clinical investigations, it is recommended that the *WHO Classification of Tumours* be used for classification and definition of tumour types and that the ICD-O code be used for storage and retrieval of data.

---

[19] *SNOMED International: The systematized nomenclature of human and veterinary medicine*. Northfield, 111: College of American Pathologists, http://www.cap.org.

HEAD AND NECK TUMOURS

Introductory Notes

The following sites are included:

- Lip, Oral cavity
- Pharynx: Oropharynx, Nasopharynx, Hypopharynx
- Larynx
- Maxillary sinus
- Nasal cavity and Ethmoid sinus
- Mucosal Malignant Melanoma
- Major Salivary glands
- Thyroid gland

Carcinomas arising in minor salivary glands of the upper aerodigestive tract are classified according to the rules for tumours of their anatomic site of origin, e.g., oral cavity.

Each site is described under the following headings:

- Rules for classification with the procedures for assessing T, N, and M categories; additional methods may be used when they enhance the accuracy of appraisal before treatment
- Anatomical sites and subsites where appropriate
- Definition of the regional lymph nodes
- TNM Clinical classification
- pTNM Pathological classification
- G Histopathological grading
- Stage grouping
- Summary

Regional Lymph Nodes

The definitions of the N categories for all head and neck sites except nasopharynx and thyroid are the same.

Midline nodes are considered ipsilateral nodes except in the thyroid.

Distant Metastasis

The definitions of the M categories for all head and neck sites are the same.

The categories M1 and pM1 may be further specified according to the following notation:

Pulmonary	PUL	Bone marrow	MAR
Osseous	OSS	Pleura	PLE
Hepatic	HEP	Peritoneum	PER
Brain	BRA	Adrenals	ADR
Lymph nodes	LYM	Skin	SKI
Others	OTH		

Histopathological Grading

The definitions of the G categories apply to all head and neck sites except thyroid and mucosal malignant melanoma. These are:

G – Histopathological Grading

GX   Grade of differentiation cannot be assessed
G1   Well differentiated
G2   Moderately differentiated
G3   Poorly differentiated
G4   Undifferentiated

R Classification

See Introduction, page 19.

Lip and Oral Cavity
(ICD-O C00, C02–06)

Rules for Classification

The classification applies to carcinomas of the vermilion surfaces of the lips and of the oral cavity, including those of minor salivary glands.

There should be histological confirmation of the disease.

The following are the procedures for assessing T, N, and M categories:

T categories	Physical examination and imaging
N categories	Physical examination and imaging
M categories	Physical examination and imaging

Anatomical Sites and Subsites

Lip (C00)
1. External upper lip (vermilion border) (C00.0)
2. External lower lip (vermilion border) (C00.1)
3. Commissures (C00.6)

Oral Cavity (C02–06)
1. Buccal mucosa
    (i)   Mucosa of upper and lower lips (C0.3, 4)
    (ii) Cheek mucosa (C06.0)

(iii) Retromolar areas (C06.2)
(iv) Bucco-alveolar sulci, upper and lower (vestibule of mouth) (C06.1)
2. Upper alveolus and gingiva (upper gum) (C03.0)
3. Lower alveolus and gingiva (lower gum) (C03.1)
4. Hard palate (C05.0)
5. Tongue
(i) Dorsal surface and lateral borders anterior to vallate papillae (anterior two-thirds) (C02.0, 1)
(ii) Inferior (ventral) surface (C02.2)
6. Floor of mouth (C04)

Regional Lymph Nodes

The regional lymph nodes are the cervical nodes.

TNM Clinical Classification

T – Primary Tumour

TX Primary tumour cannot be assessed
T0 No evidence of primary tumour
Tis Carcinoma in situ

T1 Tumour 2 cm or less in greatest dimension
T2 Tumour more than 2 cm but not more than 4 cm in greatest dimension
T3 Tumour more than 4 cm in greatest dimension
T4a *(lip)* Tumour invades through cortical bone, inferior alveolar nerve, floor of mouth, or skin (chin or nose)
T4a *(oral cavity)* Tumour invades through cortical bone, into deep/extrinsic muscle of tongue

(genioglossus, hyoglossus, palatoglossus, and styloglossus), maxillary sinus, or skin of face

T4b   *(lip and oral cavity)* Tumour invades masticator space, pterygoid plates, or skull base, or encases internal carotid artery

Note: Superficial erosion alone of bone/tooth socket by gingival primary is not sufficient to classify a tumour as T4.

N – Regional Lymph Nodes

NX   Regional lymph nodes cannot be assessed
N0   No regional lymph node metastasis
N1   Metastasis in a single ipsilateral lymph node, 3 cm or less in greatest dimension
N2   Metastasis as described below:

N2a   Metastasis in a single ipsilateral lymph node, more than 3 cm but not more than 6 cm in greatest dimension
N2b   Metastasis in multiple ipsilateral lymph nodes, none more than 6 cm in greatest dimension
N2c   Metastasis in bilateral or contralateral lymph nodes, none more than 6 cm in greatest dimension

N3   Metastasis in a lymph node more than 6 cm in greatest dimension

Note: Midline nodes are considered ipsilateral nodes.

M – Distant Metastasis

M0   No distant metastasis
M1   Distant metastasis

pTNM Pathological Classification

The pT and pN categories correspond to the T and N categories. For pM see page 15.

pN0   Histological examination of a selective neck dissection specimen will ordinarily include 6 or more lymph nodes. Histological examination of a radical or modified radical neck dissection specimen will ordinarily include 10 or more lymph nodes.

If the lymph nodes are negative, but the number ordinarily examined is not met, classify as pN0.

When size is a criterion for pN classification, measurement is made of the metastasis, not of the entire lymph node.

G Histopathological Grading

See definitions on page 24.

Stage Grouping

Stage 0	Tis	N0	M0
Stage I	T1	N0	M0
Stage II	T2	N0	M0
Stage III	T3	N0	M0
	T1, T2, T3	N1	M0
Stage IVA	T4a	N0, N1	M0
	T1, T2, T3, T4a	N2	M0
Stage IVB	Any T	N3	M0
	T4b	Any N	M0
Stage IVC	Any T	Any N	M1

Summary

Lip, Oral cavity	
T1	≤2 cm
T2	>2–4 cm
T3	>4 cm
T4a	*Lip*: through cortical bone, inferior alveolar nerve, floor of mouth, skin *Oral cavity*: through cortical bone, deep/extrinsic muscle of tongue, maxillary sinus, skin of face
T4b	Masticator space, pterygoid plates, skull base, internal carotid artery
N1	Ipsilateral single ≤3 cm
N2	(a) Ipsilateral single >3–6 cm (b) Ipsilateral multiple ≤6 cm (c) Bilateral, contralateral ≤6 cm
N3	>6 cm

Pharynx
(ICD-O C01, C05.1, 2, C09, C10.0, 2, 3, C11–13)

Rules for Classification

The classification applies to carcinomas. There should be histological confirmation of the disease.
  The following are the procedures for assessing T, N, and M categories:

T categories	Physical examination, endoscopy, and imaging
N categories	Physical examination and imaging
M categories	Physical examination and imaging

Anatomical Sites and Subsites

Oropharynx (C01, C05.1, 2, C09.0, 1, 9, C10.0, 2, 3)
1. Anterior wall (glosso-epiglottic area)
    (i)   Base of tongue (posterior to the vallate papillae or posterior third) (C01)
    (ii)   Vallecula (C10.0)
2. Lateral wall (C10.2)
    (i)   Tonsil (C09.9)
    (ii)   Tonsillar fossa (C09.0) and tonsillar (faucial) pillars (C09.1)
    (iii) Glossotonsillar sulci (tonsillar pillars) (C09.1)

3. Posterior wall (C10.3)
4. Superior wall
    (i) Inferior surface of soft palate (C05.1)
    (ii) Uvula (C05.2)

Nasopharynx (C11)

1. Postero-superior wall: extends from the level of the junction of the hard and soft palates to the base of the skull (C11.0, 1)
2. Lateral wall: including the fossa of Rosenmüller (C11.2)
3. Inferior wall: consists of the superior surface of the soft palate (C11.3)

Note: The margin of the choanal orifices, including the posterior margin of the nasal septum, is included with the nasal fossa.

Hypopharynx (C12, C13)

1. Pharyngo-oesophageal junction (postcricoid area) (C13.0): extends from the level of the arytenoid cartilages and connecting folds to the inferior border of the cricoid cartilage, thus forming the anterior wall of the hypopharynx
2. Piriform sinus (C12.9): extends from the pharyngo-epiglottic fold to the upper end of the oesophagus. It is bounded laterally by the thyroid cartilage and medially by the hypopharyngeal surface of the aryepiglottic fold (C13.1) and the arytenoid and cricoid cartilages
3. Posterior pharyngeal wall (C13.2): extends from the superior level of the hyoid bone (or floor of the vallecula) to the level of the inferior border of the cricoid cartilage and from the apex of one piriform sinus to the other

Regional Lymph Nodes

The regional lymph nodes are the cervical nodes.

The supraclavicular fossa (relevant to classifying nasopharyngeal carcinoma) is the triangular region defined by three points:

1. The superior margin of the sternal end of the clavicle
2. The superior margin of the lateral end of the clavicle
3. The point where the neck meets the shoulder. This includes caudal portions of Levels IV and V

TNM Clinical Classification

T – Primary Tumour

TX   Primary tumour cannot be assessed
T0   No evidence of primary tumour
Tis   Carcinoma in situ

Oropharynx

T1   Tumour 2 cm or less in greatest dimension
T2   Tumour more than 2 cm but not more than 4 cm in greatest dimension
T3   Tumour more than 4 cm in greatest dimension or extension to lingual surface of epiglottis
T4a   Tumour invades any of the following: larynx, deep/extrinsic muscle of tongue (genioglossus, hyoglossus, palatoglossus, and styloglossus), medial pterygoid, hard palate, or mandible*

T4b Tumour invades any of the following: lateral pterygoid muscle, pterygoid plates, lateral nasopharynx, skull base; or encases carotid artery

Note: *Mucosal extension to lingual surface of epiglottis from primary tumours of the base of the tongue and vallecula does not constitute invasion of the larynx.

Nasopharynx

T1 Tumour confined to nasopharynx, or extends to oropharynx and/or nasal cavity

T2 Tumour with parapharyngeal extension*

T3 Tumour invades bony structures of skull base and/or paranasal sinuses

T4 Tumour with intracranial extension and/or involvement of cranial nerves, hypopharynx, orbit, or with extension to the infratemporal fossa/masticator space

Note: *Parapharyngeal extension denotes postero-lateral infiltration of tumour.

Hypopharynx

T1 Tumour limited to one subsite of hypopharynx (see page 31) and/or 2 cm or less in greatest dimension

T2 Tumour invades more than one subsite of hypopharynx or an adjacent site, or measures more than 2 cm but not more than 4 cm in greatest dimension, *without* fixation of hemilarynx

T3 Tumour more than 4 cm in greatest dimension, or *with* fixation of hemilarynx or extension to oesophagus

T4a Tumour invades any of the following: thyroid/cricoid cartilage, hyoid bone, thyroid gland, oesophagus, central compartment soft tissue*

T4b   Tumour invades prevertebral fascia, encases carotid artery, or invades mediastinal structures

Note: *Central compartment soft tissue includes prelaryngeal strap muscles and subcutaneous fat.

N – Regional Lymph Nodes (*Oro- and Hypopharynx*)

NX   Regional lymph nodes cannot be assessed
N0   No regional lymph node metastasis
N1   Metastasis in a single ipsilateral lymph node, 3 cm or less in greatest dimension
N2   Metastasis as described below:
   N2a   Metastasis in a single ipsilateral lymph node, more than 3 cm but not more than 6 cm in greatest dimension
   N2b   Metastasis in multiple ipsilateral lymph nodes, none more than 6 cm in greatest dimension
   N2c   Metastasis in bilateral or contralateral lymph nodes, none more than 6 cm in greatest dimension
N3   Metastasis in a lymph node more than 6 cm in greatest dimension

Note: Midline nodes are considered ipsilateral nodes.

N – Regional Lymph Nodes (*Nasopharynx*)

NX   Regional lymph nodes cannot be assessed
N0   No regional lymph node metastasis
N1   Unilateral metastasis, in cervical lymph node(s), and/or unilateral or bilateral metastasis in retropharyngeal lymph nodes, 6 cm or less in greatest dimension, above the supraclavicular fossa

N2   Bilateral metastasis in cervical lymph node(s), 6 cm or less in greatest dimension, above the supraclavicular fossa

N3   Metastasis in cervical lymph node(s) greater than 6 cm in dimension or in the supraclavicular fossa

      N3a greater than 6 cm in dimension

      N3b extension in the supraclavicular fossa

Note: Midline nodes are considered ipsilateral nodes.

M – Distant Metastasis

M0   No distant metastasis

M1   Distant metastasis

pTNM Pathological Classification

The pT and pN categories correspond to the T and N categories. For pM see page 15.

pN0   Histological examination of a selective neck dissection specimen will ordinarily include 6 or more lymph nodes. Histological examination of a radical or modified radical neck dissection specimen will ordinarily include 10 or more lymph nodes.

      If the lymph nodes are negative, but the number ordinarily examined is not met, classify as pN0.

      When size is a criterion for pN classification, measurement is made of the metastasis, not of the entire lymph node.

G Histopathological Grading

See definitions on page 24.

Stage Grouping (Oropharynx and Hypopharynx)

Stage 0	Tis	N0	M0
Stage I	T1	N0	M0
Stage II	T2	N0	M0
Stage III	T3	N0	M0
	T1, T2, T3	N1	M0
Stage IVA	T1, T2, T3	N2	M0
	T4a	N0, N1, N2	M0
Stage IVB	T4b	Any N	M0
	Any T	N3	M0
Stage IVC	Any T	Any N	M1

Stage Grouping (Nasopharynx)

Stage 0	Tis	N0	M0
Stage I	T1	N0	M0
Stage II	T1	N1	M0
	T2	N0, N1	M0
Stage III	T1, T2	N2	M0
	T3	N0, N1, N2	M0
Stage IVA	T4	N0, N1, N2	M0
Stage IVB	Any T	N3	M0
Stage IVC	Any T	Any N	M1

Summary

Pharynx

Oropharynx

T1	≤ 2 cm
T2	>2–4 cm
T3	>4 cm
T4a	Larynx, deep/extrinsic muscle of tongue, medial pterygoid, hard palate, mandible
T4b	Lateral pterygoid muscle, pterygoid plates, lateral nasopharynx, skull base, carotid artery

Hypopharynx

T1	≤ 2 cm and limited to one subsite
T2	>2–4 cm or more than one subsite
T3	>4 cm or with hemilarynx fixation
T4a	Thyroid/cricoid cartilage, hyoid bone, thyroid gland, oesophagus, central compartment soft tissue
T4b	Prevertebral fascia, carotid artery, mediastinal structures

Oropharynx and Hypopharynx

N1	Ipsilateral single ≤ 3 cm	
N2	(a)	Ipsilateral single >3–6 cm
	(b)	Ipsilateral multiple ≤ 6 cm
	(c)	Bilateral, contralateral ≤ 6 cm
N3	>6 cm	

Summary

Nasopharynx	
T1	Nasopharynx, oropharynx, or nasal cavity
T2	Parapharyngeal extension
T3	Bony structures of skull base/paranasal sinuses
T4	Intracranial, cranial nerves, hypopharynx, orbit, infratemporal fossa/masticator space
N1	Unilateral cervical, unilateral or bilateral retropharyngeal lymph nodes, above supraclavicular fossa, ≤6 cm
N2	Bilateral cervical above supraclavicular fossa, ≤6 cm
N3a	>6 cm
N3b	Supraclavicular fossa

Larynx
(ICD-O C32.0, 1, 2, C10.1)

Rules for Classification

The classification applies to carcinomas. There should be histological confirmation of the disease.

The following are the procedures for assessing T, N, and M categories:

T categories	Physical examination, laryngoscopy, and imaging
N categories	Physical examination and imaging
M categories	Physical examination and imaging

Anatomical Sites and Subsites

1. Supraglottis (C32.1)
    (i)   Suprahyoid epiglottis [including tip, lingual (anterior) (C10.1), and laryngeal surfaces]   *Epilarynx (including marginal zone)*
    (ii) Aryepiglottic fold, laryngeal aspect
    (iii) Arytenoid
    (iv) Infrahyoid epiglottis   *Supraglottis excluding epilarynx*
    (v)   Ventricular bands (false cords)
2. Glottis (C32.0)
    (i)   Vocal cords
    (ii) Anterior commissure
    (iii) Posterior commissure
3. Subglottis (C32.2)

Regional Lymph Nodes

The regional lymph nodes are the cervical nodes.

TNM Clinical Classification

T – Primary Tumour

TX   Primary tumour cannot be assessed
T0   No evidence of primary tumour
Tis   Carcinoma in situ

Supraglottis

T1   Tumour limited to one subsite of supraglottis with normal vocal cord mobility

T2   Tumour invades mucosa of more than one adjacent subsite of supraglottis or glottis or region outside the supraglottis (e.g., mucosa of base of tongue, vallecula, medial wall of piriform sinus) without fixation of the larynx

T3   Tumour limited to larynx with vocal cord fixation and/or invades any of the following: postcricoid area, pre-epiglottic space, paraglottic space, and/or inner cortex of thyroid cartilage

T4a   Tumour invades through the thyroid cartilage and/or invades tissues beyond the larynx, e.g., trachea, soft tissues of neck including deep/extrinsic muscle of tongue (genioglossus, hyoglossus, palatoglossus, and styloglossus), strap muscles, thyroid, oesophagus

T4b   Tumour invades prevertebral space, encases carotid artery, or mediastinal structures

Glottis

T1 Tumour limited to vocal cord(s) (may involve anterior or posterior commissure) with normal mobility

  T1a Tumour limited to one vocal cord

  T1b Tumour involves both vocal cords

T2 Tumour extends to supraglottis and/or subglottis, and/or with impaired vocal cord mobility

T3 Tumour limited to larynx with vocal cord fixation and/or invades paraglottic space, and/or inner cortex of the thyroid cartilage

T4a Tumour invades through the outer cortex of the thyroid cartilage, and/or invades tissues beyond the larynx, e.g., trachea, soft tissues of neck including deep/extrinsic muscle of tongue (genioglossus, hyoglossus, palatoglossus, and styloglossus), strap muscles, thyroid, oesophagus

T4b Tumour invades prevertebral space, encases carotid artery, or mediastinal structures

Subglottis

T1 Tumour limited to subglottis

T2 Tumour extends to vocal cord(s) with normal or impaired mobility

T3 Tumour limited to larynx with vocal cord fixation

T4a Tumour invades cricoid or thyroid cartilage and/or invades tissues beyond the larynx, e.g., trachea, soft tissues of neck including deep/extrinsic muscle of tongue (genioglossus, hyoglossus, palatoglossus, and styloglossus), strap muscles, thyroid, oesophagus

T4b Tumour invades prevertebral space, encases carotid artery, or mediastinal structures

N – Regional Lymph Nodes

NX   Regional lymph nodes cannot be assessed

N0   No regional lymph node metastasis

N1   Metastasis in a single ipsilateral lymph node, 3 cm or less in greatest dimension

N2   Metastasis as described below:

  N2a   Metastasis in a single ipsilateral lymph node, more than 3 cm but not more than 6 cm in greatest dimension

  N2b   Metastasis in multiple ipsilateral lymph nodes, none more than 6 cm in greatest dimension

  N2c   Metastasis in bilateral or contralateral lymph nodes, none more than 6 cm in greatest dimension

N3   Metastasis in a lymph node more than 6 cm in greatest dimension

Note: Midline nodes are considered ipsilateral nodes.

M – Distant Metastasis

M0   No distant metastasis

M1   Distant metastasis

pTNM Pathological Classification

The pT and pN categories correspond to the T and N categories. For pM see page 15.

pN0   Histological examination of a selective neck dissection specimen will ordinarily include 6 or more lymph nodes. Histological examination of a radical or modified radical neck dissection specimen will ordinarily include 10 or more lymph nodes.

If the lymph nodes are negative, but the number ordinarily examined is not met, classify as pN0.

When size is a criterion for pN classification, measurement is made of the metastasis, not of the entire lymph node.

G Histopathological Grading

See definitions on page 24.

Stage Grouping

Stage 0	Tis	N0	M0
Stage I	T1	N0	M0
Stage II	T2	N0	M0
Stage III	T1, T2	N1	M0
	T3	N0, N1	M0
Stage IVA	T4a, T4b	N0, N1	M0
	T1, T2, T3	N2	M0
Stage IVB	T4b	Any N	M0
	Any T	N3	M0
Stage IVC	Any T	Any N	M1

Summary

Larynx

Supraglottis

T1	One subsite, normal mobility
T2	Mucosa of more than one adjacent subsite of supraglottis or glottis or adjacent region outside the supraglottis; without fixation
T3	Cord fixation or invades postcricoid area, pre-epiglottic tissues, paraglottic space, thyroid cartilage erosion
T4a	Through thyroid cartilage; trachea, soft tissues of neck: deep/extrinsic muscle of tongue, strap muscles, thyroid, oesophagus
T4b	Prevertebral space, mediastinal structures, carotid artery

Glottis

T1	Limited to vocal cord(s), normal mobility
	(a) one cord
	(b) both cords
T2	Supraglottis, subglottis, impaired cord mobility
T3	Cord fixation, paraglottic space, thyroid cartilage erosion
T4a	Through thyroid cartilage; trachea, soft tissues of neck: deep/extrinsic muscle of tongue, strap muscles, thyroid, oesophagus
T4b	Prevertebral space, mediastinal structures, carotid artery

Larynx

Subglottis

T1   Limited to subglottis

T2   Extends to vocal cord(s) with normal/ impaired mobility

T3   Cord fixation

T4a Through cricoid or thyroid cartilage; trachea, deep/extrinsic muscle of tongue, strap muscles, thyroid, oesophagus

T4b Prevertebral space, mediastinal structures, carotid artery

All Sites

N1   Ipsilateral single ≤3 cm

N2   (a) Ipsilateral single >3–6 cm
     (b) Ipsilateral multiple ≤6 cm
     (c) Bilateral, contralateral ≤6 cm

N3   >6 cm

Nasal Cavity and Paranasal Sinuses
(C30.0, 31.0, 1)

Rules for Classification

The classification applies to carcinomas. There should be histological confirmation of the disease.
The following are the procedures for assessing T, N, and M categories:

T categories	Physical examination and imaging
N categories	Physical examination and imaging
M categories	Physical examination and imaging

Anatomical Sites and Subsites

- Nasal Cavity (C30.0)   Septum
                          Floor
                          Lateral wall
                          Vestibule

- Maxillary sinus (C31.0)
- Ethmoid sinus (C31.1)   Left
                           Right

Regional Lymph Nodes

The regional lymph nodes are the cervical nodes.

TNM Clinical Classification

T – Primary Tumour

TX   Primary tumour cannot be assessed
T0   No evidence of primary tumour
Tis   Carcinoma in situ

Maxillary Sinus

T1   Tumour limited to the mucosa with no erosion or destruction of bone

T2   Tumour causing bone erosion or destruction, including extension into the hard palate and/or middle nasal meatus, except extension to posterior wall of maxillary sinus and pterygoid plates

T3   Tumour invades any of the following: bone of posterior wall of maxillary sinus, subcutaneous tissues, floor or medial wall of orbit, pterygoid fossa, ethmoid sinuses

T4a   Tumour invades any of the following: anterior orbital contents, skin of cheek, pterygoid plates, infratemporal fossa, cribriform plate, sphenoid or frontal sinuses

T4b   Tumour invades any of the following: orbital apex, dura, brain, middle cranial fossa, cranial nerves other than maxillary division of trigeminal nerve (V2), nasopharynx, or clivus

Nasal Cavity and Ethmoid Sinus

T1   Tumour restricted to one subsite of nasal cavity or ethmoid sinus, with or without bony invasion

T2   Tumour involves two subsites in a single site or extends to involve an adjacent site within the nasoethmoidal complex, with or without bony invasion

T3   Tumour extends to invade the medial wall or floor of the orbit, maxillary sinus, palate, or cribriform plate

T4a   Tumour invades any of the following: anterior orbital contents, skin of nose or cheek, minimal extension to anterior cranial fossa, pterygoid plates, sphenoid or frontal sinuses

T4b   Tumour invades any of the following: orbital apex, dura, brain, middle cranial fossa, cranial nerves other than V2, nasopharynx, or clivus

N – Regional Lymph Nodes

NX   Regional lymph nodes cannot be assessed

N0   No regional lymph node metastasis

N1   Metastasis in a single ipsilateral lymph node, 3 cm or less in greatest dimension

N2   Metastasis as described below:

   N2a Metastasis in a single ipsilateral lymph node, more than 3 cm but not more than 6 cm in greatest dimension

   N2b Metastasis in multiple ipsilateral lymph nodes, none more than 6 cm in greatest dimension

   N2c Metastasis in bilateral or contralateral lymph nodes, none more than 6 cm in greatest dimension

N3   Metastasis in a lymph node more than 6 cm in greatest dimension

Note: Midline nodes are considered ipsilateral nodes.

M – Distant Metastasis

M0   No distant metastasis

M1   Distant metastasis

pTNM Pathological Classification

The pT and pN categories correspond to the T and N categories. For pM see page 15.

pN0   Histological examination of a selective neck dissection specimen will ordinarily include 6 or more lymph nodes. Histological examination of a radical or modified radical neck dissection specimen will ordinarily include 10 or more lymph nodes.

If the lymph nodes are negative, but the number ordinarily examined is not met, classify as pN0.

When size is a criterion for pN classification, measurement is made of the metastasis, not of the entire lymph node.

G Histopathological Grading

See definitions on page 24.

Stage Grouping

Stage 0	Tis	N0	M0
Stage I	T1	N0	M0
Stage II	T2	N0	M0
Stage III	T3	N0	M0
	T1, T2, T3	N1	M0
Stage IVA	T1, T2, T3	N2	M0
	T4a	N0, N1, N2	M0
Stage IVB	T4b	Any N	M0
	Any T	N3	M0
Stage IVC	Any T	Any N	M1

Summary

Nasal Cavity and Paranasal Sinuses

Maxillary Sinus

T1	Mucosa
T2	Bone erosion/destruction, hard palate, middle nasal meatus
T3	Posterior bony wall maxillary sinus, subcutaneous tissues, floor/medial wall of orbit, pterygoid fossa, ethmoid sinus
T4a	Anterior orbit, cheek skin, pterygoid plates, infratemporal fossa, cribriform plate, sphenoid/frontal sinus
T4b	Orbital apex, dura, brain, middle cranial fossa, cranial nerves other than V2, nasopharynx, clivus

Nasal Cavity and Ethmoid Sinus

T1	One subsite
T2	Two subsites or adjacent nasoethmoidal site
T3	Medial wall/floor orbit, maxillary sinus, palate, cribriform plate
T4a	Anterior orbit, skin of nose/cheek, anterior cranial fossa (minimal), pterygoid plates, sphenoid/frontal sinuses
T4b	Orbital apex, dura, brain, middle cranial fossa, cranial nerves other than V2, nasopharynx, clivus

All Sites

N1	Ipsilateral single ≤3 cm
N2	(a) Ipsilateral single >3–6 cm
	(b) Ipsilateral multiple ≤6 cm
	(c) Bilateral, contralateral ≤6 cm
N3	>6 cm

Malignant Melanoma of Upper Aerodigestive Tract
(ICD-O C00–06, 10–14, 30–32)

Rules for Classification

The classification applies to mucosal malignant melanomas of the head and neck region, i. e., of the upper aerodigestive tract. There should be histological confirmation of the disease and division of cases by site.

The following are the procedures for assessing T, N, and M categories:

T categories	Physical examination and imaging
N categories	Physical examination and imaging
M categories	Physical examination and imaging

Regional Lymph Nodes

The regional lymph nodes are those appropriate to the site of the primary tumour. See page 24.

TNM Clinical Classification

T – Primary Tumour

TX   Primary tumour cannot be assessed
T0   No evidence of primary tumour

T3   Tumour limited to the epithelium and/or sub-mucosa (mucosal disease)

T4a   Tumour invades deep soft tissue, cartilage, bone, or overlying skin

T4b   Tumour invades any of the following: brain, dura, skull base, lower cranial nerves (IX, X, XI, XII), masticator space, carotid artery, prevertebral space, mediastinal structures

Note: Mucosal melanomas are aggressive tumours, therefore T1 and T2 are omitted as are stages I and II.

N – Regional Lymph Nodes

NX   Regional lymph nodes cannot be assessed
N0   No regional lymph node metastasis
N1   Regional lymph node metastasis

M – Distant Metastasis

M0   No distant metastasis
M1   Distant metastasis

pTNM Pathological Classification

The pT and pN categories correspond to the T and N categories. For pM see page 15.

pN0 Histological examination of a regional lymphadenectomy specimen will ordinarily include 6 or more lymph nodes.

If the lymph nodes are negative, but the number ordinarily examined is not met, classify as pN0.

Stage Grouping

Stage III	T3	N0	M0
Stage IVA	T4a	N0	M0
	T3, T4a	N1	M0
Stage IVB	T4b	Any N	M0
Stage IVC	Any T	Any N	M1

Summary

Melanoma: Upper aerodigestive

T3	Epithelium/submucosa (mucosal disease)
T4a	Deep soft tissue, cartilage, bone, or overlying skin
T4b	Brain, dura, skull base, lower cranial nerves, masticator space, carotid artery, prevertebral space, mediastinal structures

Major Salivary Glands
(ICD-O C07, C08)

Rules for Classification

The classification applies to carcinomas of the major salivary glands. Tumours arising in minor salivary glands (mucus-secreting glands in the lining membrane of the upper aerodigestive tract) are not included in this classification but at their anatomic site of origin, e.g., lip. There should be histological confirmation of the disease.

The following are the procedures for assessing T, N, and M categories:

T categories	Physical examination and imaging
N categories	Physical examination and imaging
M categories	Physical examination and imaging

Anatomical Sites

- Parotid gland (C07.9)
- Submandibular (submaxillary) gland (C08.0)
- Sublingual gland (C08.1)

Regional Lymph Nodes

The regional lymph nodes are the cervical nodes.

TNM Clinical Classification

T – Primary Tumour

TX   Primary tumour cannot be assessed
T0   No evidence of primary tumour

T1   Tumour 2 cm or less in greatest dimension without extraparenchymal extension*

T2   Tumour more than 2 cm but not more than 4 cm in greatest dimension without extraparenchymal extension*

T3   Tumour more than 4 cm and/or tumour with extraparenchymal extension*

T4a   Tumour invades skin, mandible, ear canal, and/or facial nerve

T4b   Tumour invades base of skull, and/or pterygoid plates, and/or encases carotid artery

Note: *Extraparenchymal extension is clinical or macroscopic evidence of invasion of soft tissues or nerve, except those listed under T4a and 4b. Microscopic evidence alone does not constitute extraparenchymal extension for classification purposes.

N – Regional Lymph Nodes

NX   Regional lymph nodes cannot be assessed
N0   No regional lymph node metastasis
N1   Metastasis in a single ipsilateral lymph node, 3 cm or less in greatest dimension
N2   Metastasis as described below:
    N2a   Metastasis in a single ipsilateral lymph node, more than 3 cm but not more than 6 cm in greatest dimension

N2b Metastasis in multiple ipsilateral lymph nodes, none more than 6 cm in greatest dimension

N2c Metastasis in bilateral or contralateral lymph nodes, none more than 6 cm in greatest dimension

N3 Metastasis in a lymph node more than 6 cm in greatest dimension

Note: Midline nodes are considered ipsilateral nodes.

M – Distant Metastasis

M0 No distant metastasis

M1 Distant metastasis

pTNM Pathological Classification

The pT and pN categories correspond to the T and N categories. For pM see page 15.

pN0 Histological examination of a selective neck dissection specimen will ordinarily include 6 or more lymph nodes. Histological examination of a radical or modified radical neck dissection specimen will ordinarily include 10 or more lymph nodes.

If the lymph nodes are negative, but the number ordinarily examined is not met, classify as pN0.

When size is a criterion for pN classification, measurement is made of the metastasis, not of the entire lymph node.

G Histopathological Grading

See definitions on page 24.

Stage Grouping

Stage I	T1	N0	M0
Stage II	T2	N0	M0
Stage III	T3	N0	M0
	T1, T2, T3	N1	M0
Stage IVA	T4a, T4b	N0, N1	M0
	T1, T2, T3, T4a	N2	M0
Stage IVB	T4b	Any N	M0
	Any T	N3	M0
Stage IVC	Any T	Any N	M1

Summary

Salivary Glands	
T1	≤2 cm, without extraparenchymal extension
T2	>2–4 cm, without extraparenchymal extension
T3	>4 cm and/or extraparenchymal extension
T4a	Skin, mandible, ear canal, facial nerve
T4b	Skull, pterygoid plates, carotid artery
N1	Ipsilateral single ≤3 cm
N2	(a) Ipsilateral single >3–6 cm
	(b) Ipsilateral multiple ≤6 cm
	(c) Bilateral, contralateral ≤6 cm
N3	>6 cm

Thyroid Gland
(ICD-O C73)

Rules for Classification

The classification applies to carcinomas. There should be microscopic confirmation of the disease and division of cases by histological type.

The following are the procedures for assessing T, N, and M categories:

T categories	Physical examination, endoscopy, and imaging
N categories	Physical examination and imaging
M categories	Physical examination and imaging

Regional Lymph Nodes

The regional lymph nodes are the cervical and upper/superior mediastinal nodes.

TNM Clinical Classification

T – Primary Tumour

TX   Primary tumour cannot be assessed
T0   No evidence of primary tumour

T1   Tumour 2 cm or less in greatest dimension, limited to the thyroid

T1a Tumour 1 cm or less in greatest dimension, limited to the thyroid

T1b Tumour more than 1 cm but not more than 2 cm in greatest dimension, limited to the thyroid

T2 Tumour more than 2 cm but not more than 4 cm in greatest dimension, limited to the thyroid

T3 Tumour more than 4 cm in greatest dimension, limited to the thyroid or any tumour with minimal extrathyroid extension (e.g., extension to sternothyroid muscle or perithyroid soft tissues)

T4a Tumour extends beyond the thyroid capsule and invades any of the following: subcutaneous soft tissues, larynx, trachea, oesophagus, recurrent laryngeal nerve

T4b Tumour invades prevertebral fascia, mediastinal vessels, or encases carotid artery

All anaplastic carcinomas are considered T4 tumours

T4a* (anaplastic carcinoma only) Tumour (any size) limited to the thyroid

T4b* (anaplastic carcinoma only) Tumour (any size) extends beyond the thyroid capsules

Notes: Multifocal tumours of all histological types should be designated (m) (the largest determines the classification), e.g., T2(m).

N – Regional Lymph Nodes

NX Regional lymph nodes cannot be assessed

N0 No regional lymph node metastasis

N1 Regional lymph node metastasis
    N1a Metastasis in Level VI (pretracheal, para-tracheal, and prelaryngeal/Delphian lymph nodes)
    N1b Metastasis in other unilateral, bilateral or contralateral cervical (Levels I, II II, IV, or V) or retropharyngeal or superior mediastinal lymph nodes

M – Distant Metastasis

M0 No distant metastasis
M1 Distant metastasis

pTNM Pathological Classification

The pT and pN categories correspond to the T and N categories. For pM see page 15.

pN0 Histological examination of a selective neck dissection specimen will ordinarily include 6 or more lymph nodes. If the lymph nodes are negative, but the number ordinarily examined is not met, classify as pN0.

Histopathological Types

The four major histopathological types are:

- Papillary carcinoma (including those with follicular foci)
- Follicular carcinoma (including so-called Hürthle cell carcinoma)
- Medullary carcinoma
- Anaplastic/undifferentiated carcinoma

Stage Grouping

Separate stage groupings are recommended for papillary and follicular (differentiated), medullary, and anaplastic (undifferentiated) carcinomas:

Papillary or Follicular

Under 45 years

Stage I	Any T	Any N	M0
Stage II	Any T	Any N	M1

Papillary or Follicular *45 years and older*

Stage I	T1a, T1b	N0	M0
Stage II	T2	N0	M0
Stage III	T3	N0	M0
	T1, T2, T3	N1a	M0
Stage IVA	T1, T2, T3	N1b	M0
	T4a	N0, N1	M0
Stage IVB	T4b	Any N	M0
Stage IVC	Any T	Any N	M1

Medullary

Stage I	T1a, T1b	N0	M0
Stage II	T2, T3	N0	M0
Stage III	T1, T2, T3	N1a	M0
Stage IVA	T1, T2, T3	N1b	M0
	T4a	Any N	M0
Stage IVB	T4b	Any N	M0
Stage IVC	Any T	Any N	M1

Anaplastic Carcinoma
All anaplastic carcinoma are stage IV

Stage IVA	T4a	Any N	M0
Stage IVB	T4b	Any N	M0
Stage IVC	Any T	Any N	M1

Summary

Thyroid Gland

Papillary, follicular, and medullary carcinoma

T1	≤2 cm, intrathyroidal
T2	>2–4 cm, intrathyroidal
T3	>4 cm or minimal extrathyroidal extension
T4a	Subcutaneous, larynx, trachea, oesophagus, recurrent laryngeal nerve
T4b	Prevertebral fascia, mediastinal vessels, carotid artery

Anaplastic/undifferentiated carcinoma

T4a	Tumour limited to thyroid
T4b	Tumour beyond thyroid capsule

All types

N1a	Level VI
N1b	Other regional

DIGESTIVE SYSTEM TUMOURS

The following sites are included:

- Oesophagus and Oesophagogastric junction
- Stomach
- Gastrointestinal stromal tumour (GIST)
- Small Intestine
- Carcinoid (neuroendocrine) tumours
- Appendix
- Colon and Rectum
- Anal canal
- Liver cell carcinoma
- Intrahepatic cholangiocarcinoma
- Gallbladder
- Perihilar bile duct; distal extrahepatic bile duct
- Ampulla of Vater
- Pancreas

Each site is described under the following headings:

- Rules for classification with the procedures for assessing T, N, and M categories; additional methods may be used when they enhance the accuracy of appraisal before treatment
- Anatomical sites and subsites where appropriate
- Definition of the regional lymph nodes

- TNM Clinical classification
- pTNM Pathological classification
- G Histopathological grading
- Stage grouping
- Summary

Regional Lymph Nodes

The number of lymph nodes ordinarily included in a lymphadenectomy specimen is noted at each site.

Distant Metastasis

The categories M1 and pM1 may be further specified according to the following notation:

Pulmonary	PUL	Bone marrow	MAR
Osseous	OS S	Pleura	PLE
Hepatic	HEP	Peritoneum	PER
Brain	BRA	Adrenals	ADR
Lymph nodes	LYM	Skin	SKI
Others	OTH		

Histopathological Grading

The definitions of the G categories apply to all digestive system tumours except liver. These are:

G — Histopathological Grading

GX   Grade of differentiation cannot be assessed
G1   Well differentiated
G2   Moderately differentiated
G3   Poorly differentiated
G4   Undifferentiated

R Classification

See Introduction, page 19.

Oesophagus including Oesophagogastric Junction
(ICD-O C15)

Includes Oesophagogastric Junction (C16.0)

Rules for Classification

The classification applies to carcinomas and includes adenocarcinomas of the oesophagogastric junction. There should be histological confirmation of the disease and division of cases by topographic localization and histological type. A tumour the epicentre of which is within 5 cm of the *oesophagogastric junction* and also extends into the oesophagus is classified and staged using the oesophageal scheme. Tumours with an epicentre in the stomach greater than 5 cm from the oesophagogastric junction or those within 5 cm of the oesophagogastric junction without extension in the oesophagus are classified and staged using the gastric carcinoma scheme.

The following are the procedures for assessing T, N, and M categories:

T categories	Physical examination, imaging, endoscopy (including bronchoscopy), and/or surgical exploration

| N categories | Physical examination, imaging, and/or surgical exploration |
| M categories | Physical examination, imaging, and/or surgical exploration |

Anatomical Subsites

1. Cervical oesophagus (C15.0): this commences at the lower border of the cricoid cartilage and ends at the thoracic inlet (suprasternal notch), approximately 18 cm from the upper incisor teeth.
2. Intrathoracic oesophagus
   (i) The upper thoracic portion (C15.3) extending from the thoracic inlet to the level of the tracheal bifurcation, approximately 24 cm from the upper incisor teeth
   (ii) The mid-thoracic portion (C15.4) is the proximal half of the oesophagus between the tracheal bifurcation and the oesophagogastric junction. The lower level is approximately 32 cm from the upper incisor teeth.
   (iii) The lower thoracic portion (C15.5), approximately 8 cm in length (includes abdominal oesophagus), is the distal half of the oesophagus between the tracheal bifurcation and the oesophagogastric junction. The lower level is approximately 40 cm from the upper incisor teeth.
3. Oesophagogastric junction (C16.0)

Regional Lymph Nodes

The regional lymph nodes, irrespective of the site of the primary tumour, are those in the oesophageal drainage area including coeliac axis nodes and paraesophageal nodes in the neck, but not supraclavicular nodes.

TNM Clinical Classification

T – Primary Tumour

TX   Primary tumour cannot be assessed
T0   No evidence of primary tumour
Tis   Carcinoma in situ/high-grade dysplasia

T1   Tumour invades lamina propria, muscularis mucosae, or submucosa
       T1a Tumour invades lamina propria or muscularis mucosae
       T1b Tumour invades submucosa
T2   Tumour invades muscularis propria
T3   Tumour invades adventitia
T4   Tumour invades adjacent structures
       T4a Tumour invades pleura, pericardium, or diaphragm
       T4b Tumour invades other adjacent structures such as aorta, vertebral body, or trachea

N – Regional Lymph Nodes

NX   Regional lymph nodes cannot be assessed
N0   No regional lymph node metastasis
N1   Metastasis in 1–2 regional lymph nodes
N2   Metastasis in 3–6 regional lymph nodes
N3   Metastasis in 7 or more regional lymph nodes

M – Distant Metastasis

M0   No distant metastasis
M1   Distant metastasis

pTNM Pathological Classification

The pT and pN categories correspond to the T and N categories. For pM see page 15.

pN0   Histological examination of a regional lymph-adenectomy specimen will ordinarily include 6 or more lymph nodes.

        If the lymph nodes are negative, but the number ordinarily examined is not met, classify as pN0.

G Histopathological Grading

See definitions on page 65.

Stage Grouping

Carcinomas of the oesophagus and oesophagogastric junction

Stage	T	N	M
Stage 0	Tis	N0	M0
Stage IA	T1	N0	M0
Stage IB	T2	N0	M0
Stage IIA	T3	N0	M0
Stage IIB	T1, T2	N1	M0
Stage IIIA	T4a	N0	M0
	T3	N1	M0
	T1, T2	N2	M0
Stage IIIB	T3	N2	M0
Stage IIIC	T4a	N1, N2	M0
	T4b	Any N	M0
	Any T	N3	M0
Stage IV	Any T	Any N	M1

Prognostic Grouping

Squamous Cell Carcinoma

	T	N	M	Grade	Location*
Group 0	Tis	0	0	1	Any
Group IA	1	0	0	1, X	Any
Group IB	1	0	0	2, 3	Any
	2, 3	0	0	1, X	Lower, X
Group IIA	2, 3	0	0	1, X	Upper, middle
	2, 3	0	0	2, 3	Lower, X
Group IIB	2, 3	0	0	2, 3	Upper, middle
	1, 2	1	0	Any	Any
Group IIIA	1, 2	2	0	Any	Any
	3	1	0	Any	Any
	4a	0	0	Any	Any
Group IIIB	3	2	0	Any	Any
Group IIIC	4a	1, 2	0	Any	Any
	4b	Any	0	Any	Any
	Any	3	0	Any	Any
Group IV	Any	Any	1	Any	Any

Note: *Lower, middle and upper correspond to the intrathoracic thirds of the oesophagus

Adenocarcinoma

	T	N	M	Grade
Group 0	Tis	0	0	1
Group IA	1	0	0	1, 2, X
Group IB	1	0	0	3
	2	0	0	1, 2, X
Group IIA	2	0	0	3
Group IIB	3	0	0	Any
	1, 2	1	0	Any
Group IIIA	1, 2	2	0	Any
	3	1	0	Any
	4a	0	0	Any
Group IIIB	3	2	0	Any
Group IIIC	4a	1, 2	0	Any
	4b	Any	0	Any
	Any	3	0	Any
Group IV	Any	Any	1	Any

Summary

Oesophagus (includes oesophagogastric junction)

T1	Lamina propria (T1a), submucosa (T1b)
T2	Muscularis propria
T3	Adventitia
T4a	Pleura, pericardium, diaphragm
T4b	Aorta, vertebral body, trachea
N1	1–2 regional
N2	3–6 regional
N3	7 or more regional
M1	Distant metastasis

Stomach
(ICD-O C16)

Rules for Classification

The classification applies to carcinomas. There should be histological confirmation of the disease. A tumour the epicentre of which is within 5 cm of the *oesophagogastric junction* and also extends into the oesophagus is classified and staged according to the oesophageal scheme. All other tumours with an epicentre in the stomach greater than 5 cm from the oesophagogastric junction, or those within 5 cm of the junction without extension into the oesophagus, are staged using the gastric carcinoma scheme.

The following are the procedures for assessing T, N, and M categories:

T categories	Physical examination, imaging, endoscopy, and/or surgical exploration
N categories	Physical examination, imaging, and/or surgical exploration
M categories	Physical examination, imaging, and/or surgical exploration

Anatomical Subsites

1. Fundus (C16.1)
2. Corpus (C16.2)
3. Antrum (C16.3) and pylorus (C16.4)

Regional Lymph Nodes

The regional lymph nodes of the stomach are the perigastric nodes along the lesser and greater curvatures, the nodes along the left gastric, common hepatic, splenic, and coeliac arteries, and the hepatoduodenal nodes.

Involvement of other intra-abdominal lymph nodes such as retropancreatic, mesenteric, and para-aortic is classified as distant metastasis.

TNM Clinical Classification

T – Primary Tumour

TX   Primary tumour cannot be assessed
T0   No evidence of primary tumour
Tis   Carcinoma in situ: intraepithelial tumour without invasion of the lamina propria, high grade dysplasia

T1   Tumour invades lamina propria, muscularis mucosae, or submucosa
        T1a Tumour invades lamina propria or muscularis mucosae
        T1b Tumour invades submucosa
T2   Tumour invades muscularis propria
T3   Tumour invades subserosa

T4   Tumour perforates serosa or invades adjacent structures[1, 2, 3]

T4a   Tumour perforates serosa

T4b   Tumour invades adjacent structures[1, 2, 3]

Notes: 1. The adjacent structures of the stomach are the spleen, transverse colon, liver, diaphragm, pancreas, abdominal wall, adrenal gland, kidney, small intestine, and retroperitoneum.
2. Intramural extension to the duodenum or oesophagus is classified by the depth of greatest invasion in any of these sites, including stomach.
3. Tumour that extends into gastrocolic or gastrohepatic ligaments or into greater or lesser omentum, without perforation of visceral peritoneum, is T3.

N – Regional Lymph Nodes

NX   Regional lymph nodes cannot be assessed

N0   No regional lymph node metastasis

N1   Metastasis in 1 to 2 regional lymph nodes

N2   Metastasis in 3 to 6 regional lymph nodes

N3   Metastasis in 7 or more regional lymph nodes

N3a   Metastasis in 7–15 regional lymph nodes

N3b   Metastasis in 16 or more regional lymph nodes

M – Distant Metastasis

M0   No distant metastasis

M1   Distant metastasis

Note: Distant metastasis includes peritoneal seeding, positive peritoneal cytology, and omental tumour not part of continuous extension.

pTNM Pathological Classification

The pT and pN categories correspond to the T and N categories. For pM see page 15.

pN0   Histological examination of a regional lymphadenectomy specimen will ordinarily include 16 or more lymph nodes.

If the lymph nodes are negative, but the number ordinarily examined is not met, classify as pN0.

G Histopathological Grading

See definitions on page 65.

Stage Grouping

Stage 0	Tis	N0	M0
Stage IA	T1	N0	M0
Stage IB	T2	N0	M0
	T1	N1	M0
Stage IIA	T3	N0	M0
	T2	N1	M0
	T1	N2	M0
Stage IIB	T4a	N0	M0
	T3	N1	M0
	T2	N2	M0
	T1	N3	M0
Stage IIIA	T4a	N1	M0
	T3	N2	M0
	T2	N3	M0
Stage IIIB	T4b	N0, N1	M0
	T4a	N2	M0
	T3	N3	M0
Stage IIIC	T4a	N3	M0
	T4b	N2, N3	M0
Stage IV	Any T	Any N	M1

Summary

Stomach	
T1	Lamina propria (T1a), submucosa (T1b)
T2	Muscularis propria
T3	Subserosa
T4a	Perforates serosa
T4b	Adjacent structures
N1	1–2 nodes
N2	3–6 nodes
N3a	7–15 nodes
N3b	16 or more

Gastrointestinal Stromal Tumour (GIST)

Rules for Classification

The classification applies to gastrointestinal stromal tumours. There should be histological confirmation of the disease.

The following are the procedures for assessing the T, N, and M categories:

T categories	Physical examination, imaging, endoscopy, and/or surgical exploration
N categories	Physical examination, imaging, and/or surgical exploration
M categories	Physical examination, imaging, and/or surgical exploration

Anatomical Sites and Subsites

- Oesophagus (C15)
- Stomach (C16)
- Small intestine (C17)
  1. Duodenum (C17.0)
  2. Jejunum (C17.1)
  3. Ileum (C17.2)

- Colon (C18)
- Rectum (C20)
- Omentum (C48.1)
- Mesentery (C48.1)

Regional Lymph Nodes

The regional lymph nodes are those appropriate to the site of the primary tumour; see gastrointestinal sites for details.

TNM Clinical Classification

T – Primary Tumour

TX   Primary tumour cannot be assessed
T0   No evidence for primary tumour

T1   Tumour 2 cm or less
T2   Tumour more than 2 cm but not more than 5 cm in greatest dimension
T3   Tumour more than 5 cm but not more than 10 cm in greatest dimension
T4   Tumour more than 10 cm in greatest dimension

N – Regional Lymph Nodes

NX   Regional lymph nodes cannot be assessed*
N0   No regional lymph node metastasis
N1   Regional lymph node metastasis

Note: *NX: Regional lymph node involvement is rare for GISTs, so that cases in which the nodal status is not assessed clinically or pathologically could be considered N0 instead of NX or pNX.

M – Distant Metastasis

M0   No distant metastasis
M1   Distant metastasis

pTNM Pathological Classification

The pT and pN categories correspond to the T and N categories. For pM see page 15.

G Histopathological Grading

Grading for GIST is dependent on mitotic rate.*
    Low mitotic rate: 5 or fewer per 50 hpf
    High mitotic rate: over 5 per 50 hpf

Note: *The mitotic rate of GIST is best expressed as the number of mitoses per 50 high power fields (hpf) using the 40X objective (total area 5 mm^2 in 50 fields)

Stage Grouping

Gastric GIST*

				Mitotic rate
Stage IA	T1, T2	N0	M0	Low
Stage IB	T3	N0	M0	Low
Stage II	T1, T2	N0	M0	High
	T4	N0	M0	Low
Stage IIIA	T3	N0	M0	High
Stage IIIB	T4	N0	M0	High
Stage IV	Any T	N1	M0	Any rate
	Any T	Any N	M1	Any rate

Small Intestinal GIST*

				Mitotic rate
Stage I	T1, T2	N0	M0	Low
Stage II	T3	N0	M0	Low
Stage IIIA	T1	N0	M0	High
	T4	N0	M0	Low
Stage IIIB	T2, T3, T4	N0	M0	High
Stage IV	Any T	N1	M0	Any rate
	Any T	Any N	M1	Any rate

Note: *Staging criteria for gastric tumours can be applied in primary, solitary omental GISTs. Staging criteria for intestinal tumours can be applied to GISTs in less common sites, such as oesophagus, colon, rectum, and mesentery.

Summary

Gastrointestinal Stromal Tumour	
T1	≤2 cm
T2	>2 cm to 5 cm
T3	>5 cm to 10 cm
T4	>10 cm

Small Intestine
(ICD-O C17)

Rules for Classification

The classification applies to carcinomas. There should be histological confirmation of the disease.

The following are the procedures for assessing T, N, and M categories:

T categories	Physical examination, imaging, endoscopy, and/or surgical exploration
N categories	Physical examination, imaging, and/or surgical exploration
M categories	Physical examination, imaging, and/or surgical exploration

Anatomical Subsites

1. Duodenum (C17.0)
2. Jejunum (C17.1)
3. Ileum (C17.2) (excludes ileocaecal valve C18.0)

Note: This classification does not apply to carcinomas of the ampulla of Vater (see page 129).

Regional Lymph Nodes

The regional lymph nodes for the duodenum are the pancreaticoduodenal, pyloric, hepatic (pericholedochal, cystic, hilar), and superior mesenteric nodes.

The regional lymph nodes for the ileum and jejunum are the mesenteric nodes, including the superior mesenteric nodes, and, for the terminal ileum only, the ileocolic nodes including the posterior caecal nodes.

TNM Clinical Classification

T – Primary Tumour

TX   Primary tumour cannot be assessed
T0   No evidence of primary tumour
Tis   Carcinoma in situ

T1   Tumour invades lamina propria, muscularis mucosae or submucosa
       T1a   Tumour invades lamina propria or muscularis mucosae
       T1b   Tumour invades submucosa
T2   Tumour invades muscularis propria
T3   Tumour invades subserosa or non-peritonealized perimuscular tissue (mesentery or retroperitoneum*) with extension 2 cm or less
T4   Tumour perforates visceral peritoneum or directly invades other organs or structures (includes other loops of small intestine, mesentery, or retroperitoneum more than 2 cm and abdominal wall by way of serosa; for duodenum only, invasion of pancreas)

Note: *The non-peritonealized perimuscular tissue is, for jejunum and ileum, part of the mesentery and, for duodenum in areas where serosa is lacking, part of the retroperitoneum.

N – Regional Lymph Nodes

NX   Regional lymph nodes cannot be assessed
N0   No regional lymph node metastasis
N1   Metastasis in 1–3 regional lymph nodes
N2   Metastasis in 4 or more regional lymph nodes

M – Distant Metastasis

M0   No distant metastasis
M1   Distant metastasis

pTNM Pathological Classification

The pT and pN categories correspond to the T and N categories. For pM see page 15.

pN0   Histological examination of a regional lymph-adenectomy specimen will ordinarily include 6 or more lymph nodes.

If the lymph nodes are negative, but the number ordinarily examined is not met, classify as pN0.

G Histopathological Grading

See definitions on page 65.

Stage Grouping

Stage 0	Tis	N0	M0
Stage I	T1, T2	N0	M0
Stage IIA	T3	N0	M0
Stage IIB	T4	N0	M0
Stage IIIA	Any T	N1	M0
Stage IIIB	Any T	N2	M0
Stage IV	Any T	Any N	M1

Summary

Small Intestine

T1	Lamina propria, submucosa
T2	Muscularis propria
T3	Subserosa, non-peritonealized perimuscular tissues (mesentery, retroperitoneum) ≤ 2 cm
T4	Visceral peritoneum, other organs/structures including mesentery, retroperitoneum >2 cm
N1	1 to 3 nodes
N2	$>$ 3 nodes

Appendix - Carcinoma
(ICD-O C18.1)

Rules for Classification

This section includes two separate classifications: one for carcinoma and one for carcinoid. There should be histological confirmation of the disease and separation of carcinomas into mucinous and non-mucinous adenocarcinomas.

Goblet cell carcinoids are classified according to the carcinoma scheme.

Grading is of particular importance for mucinous tumours.

The following are the procedures for assessing T, N, and M categories:

T categories	Physical examination, imaging, and/or surgical exploration
N categories	Physical examination, imaging, and/or surgical exploration
M categories	Physical examination, imaging, and/or surgical exploration

Anatomical Site

Appendix (C18.1)

The ileocolic are the regional lymph nodes.

Carcinoma

T – Primary Tumour

TX   Primary tumour cannot be assessed
T0   No evidence of primary tumour
Tis   Carcinoma in situ: intraepithelial or invasion of lamina propria[1]

T1   Tumour invades submucosa
T2   Tumour invades muscularis propria
T3   Tumour invades subserosa or mesoappendix
T4   Tumour perforates visceral peritoneum, including mucinous peritoneal tumour within the right lower quadrant and/or directly invades other organs or structures[2,3]

      T4a Tumour perforates visceral peritoneum, including mucinous peritoneal tumour within the right lower quadrant
      T4b Tumour directly invades other organs or structures[2,3]

Notes: 1. Tis includes cancer cells confined within the glandular basement membrane (intraepithelial) or lamina propria (intramucosal) with no extension through muscularis mucosae into submucosa.
       2. Direct invasion in T4 includes invasion of other intestinal segments by way of the serosa, e.g., invasion of ileum.

3. Tumour that is adherent to other organs or structures, macroscopically, is classified T4b. However, if no tumour is present in the adhesion, microscopically, the classification should be pT1, 2, or 3.

N – Regional Lymph Nodes

NX   Regional lymph nodes cannot be assessed
N0   No regional lymph node metastasis
N1   Metastasis in 1–3 regional lymph nodes
N2   Metastasis in 4 or more regional lymph nodes

Note: A satellite peritumoural nodule in the periappendiceal adipose tissue of a primary carcinoma without histological evidence of residual lymph node in the nodule may represent discontinuous spread (T3), venous invasion with extravascular spread (T3, V1/2) or a totally replaced lymph node (N1/2).

M – Distant Metastasis

M0   No distant metastasis
M1   Distant metastasis
     M1a Intraperitoneal metastasis beyond the right lower quadrant, including pseudomyxoma peritonei
     M1b Non-peritoneal metastasis

pTNM Pathological Classification

The pT and pN categories correspond to the T and N categories. For pM see page 15.

pN0   Histological examination of a regional lymphadenectomy specimen will ordinarily include 12 or more lymph nodes.

If the lymph nodes are negative, but the number ordinarily examined is not met, classify as pN0.

G Histopathological Grading

GX	Grade of differentiation cannot be assessed	
G1	Well differentiated	Mucinous low grade
G2	Moderately differentiated	Mucinous high grade
G3	Poorly differentiated	Mucinous high grade
G4	Undifferentiated	

Stage Grouping

Carcinoma				
Stage 0	Tis	N0	M0	
Stage I	T1, T2	N0	M0	
Stage IIA	T3	N0	M0	
IIB	T4a	N0	M0	
IIC	T4b	N0	M0	
Stage IIIA	T1, T2	N1	M0	
IIIB	T3, T4	N1	M0	
IIIC	Any T	N2	M0	
Stage IVA	Any T	N0	M1a	G1
IVB	Any T	N0	M1a	G2, G3
	Any T	N1, N2	M1a	Any G
Stage IVC	Any T	Any N	M1b	Any G

Summary

Appendix–Carcinoma:
Separate mucinous from non-mucinous
carcinomas

T1	Submucosa
T2	Muscularis propria
T3	Subserosa, non-peritonealized periappendiceal tissues, mesoappendix
T4a	Perforates visceral peritoneum/Mucinous peritoneal tumour within right lower quadrant
T4b	Other organs or structures
N1	≤3 regional
N2	>3 regional
M1a	Intraperitoneal metastasis beyond right lower quadrant, pseudomyxoma peritonei
M1b	Non-peritoneal metastasis

Appendix - Carcinoid
(Well-differentiated Neuroendocrine Tumour)

TNM Clinical Classification

T – Primary Tumour[1]

TX   Primary tumour cannot be assessed
T0   No evidence of primary tumour

T1   Tumour 2 cm or less in greatest dimension
     T1a   Tumour 1 cm or less in greatest dimension
     T1b   Tumour more than 1 cm but not more than 2 cm

T2   Tumour more than 2 cm but not more than 4 cm or with extension to the caecum

T3   Tumour more than 4 cm or with extension to the ileum

T4   Tumour perforates peritoneum or invades other adjacent organs or structures, e.g., abdominal wall and skeletal muscle [2]

Note: 1. Goblet cell carcinoid is classified according to the carcinoma scheme.
      2. Tumour that is adherent to other organs or structures, macroscopically, is classified T4. However, if no tumour is present in the adhesion, microscopically, the classification should be classified pT1–3.

N – Regional Lymph Nodes

NX   Regional lymph nodes cannot be assessed
N0   No regional lymph node metastasis
N1   Regional lymph node metastasis

M – Distant Metastasis

M0   No distant metastasis
M1   Distant metastasis

pTNM Pathological Classification

The pT and pN categories correspond to the T and N categories. For pM see page 15.

pN0   Histological examination of a regional lymphadenectomy specimen will ordinarily include 12 or more lymph nodes.

If the lymph nodes are negative, but the number ordinarily examined is not met, classify as pN0.

Histopathological Grading

Histological grading is not carried out for carcinoid tumours, but a mitotic count of 2–10 per 10 hpf and/or focal necrosis are features of atypical carcinoids, a type seen much more commonly in the lung than in the appendix.

Stage Grouping

Carcinoid			
Stage I	T1	N0	M0
Stage II	T2, T3	N0	M0
Stage III	T4	N0	M0
	Any T	N1	M0
Stage IV	Any T	Any N	M1

Summary

Appendix – Carcinoid (Well-differentiated neuroendocrine tumour)	
T1a	≤1 cm
T1b	>1–2 cm
T2	>2–4 cm; caecum
T3	>4 cm; ileum
T4	Perforates peritoneum; other organs or structures
N1	Regional

Gastric, Small & Large Intestinal Carcinoid Tumours
(Well-differentiated Neuroendocrine Tumours and Well-differentiated Neuroendocrine Carcinomas)

Rules for Classification

This classification system applies to carcinoid tumours (well-differentiated neuroendocrine tumours) and atypical carcinoid tumours (well-differentiated neuroendocrine carcinomas) of the gastrointestinal tract, excluding the appendix.

Neuroendocrine/endocrine tumours of the pancreas and lung should be classified according to criteria for carcinoma at those sites. Merkel cell carcinoma of the skin has a separate classification.

High-grade neuroendocrine carcinomas are excluded and should be classified according to criteria for classifying carcinomas at the respective site.

Regional lymph nodes

The regional lymph nodes correspond to those listed under the appropriate sites for carcinoma.

TNM Clinical Classification-Stomach

T – Primary Tumour

TX   Primary tumour cannot be assessed
T0   No evidence of primary tumour
Tis   Carcinoid in situ/dysplasia (tumour less than 0.5 mm, confined to mucosa)

T1   Tumour confined to mucosa and 0.5 mm or more but no greater than 1 cm in size; or invades submucosa and is no greater than 1 cm in greatest dimension
T2   Tumour invades muscularis propria or is more than 1 cm in greatest dimension
T3   Tumour invades subserosa
T4   Tumour perforates visceral peritoneum (serosa) or other organs or adjacent structures

Note: For any T, add (m) for multiple tumours.

N – Regional Lymph Nodes

NX   Regional lymph nodes cannot be assessed
N0   No regional lymph node metastasis
N1   Regional lymph node metastasis

M – Distant Metastasis

M0   No distant metastasis
M1   Distant metastasis

TNM Clinical Classification
Duodenum/ampulla/jejunum/ileum

T – Primary Tumour

TX   Primary tumour cannot be assessed
T0   No evidence of primary tumour

T1   Tumour invades lamina propria or submucosa and is no greater than 1 cm in size[*]
T2   Tumour invades muscularis propria or is greater than 1 cm in size
T3   Jejunal or ileal tumour invades subserosa
       Ampullary or duodenal tumour invades pancreas or retroperitoneum
T4   Tumour perforates visceral peritoneum (serosa) or invades other organs or adjacent structures

Note: [*]Tumour limited to ampulla of Vater for ampullary gangliocytic paraganglioma.
        For any T, add (m) for multiple tumours.

N – Regional Lymph Nodes

NX   Regional lymph nodes cannot be assessed
N0   No regional lymph node metastasis
N1   Regional lymph node metastasis

M – Distant Metastasis

M0   No distant metastasis
M1   Distant metastasis

TNM Clinical Classification
Large Intestine

T – Primary Tumour

TX   Primary tumour cannot be assessed
T0   No evidence of primary tumour

T1   Tumour invades lamina propria or submucosa
      and is no greater than 2 cm in size
      T1a   Tumour less than 1 cm in size
      T1b   Tumour 1–2 cm in size
T2   Tumour invades muscularis propria or is greater
      than 2 cm in size
T3   Tumour invades subserosa, or non-peritoneal-
      ized pericolic or perirectal tissues
T4   Tumour perforates peritoneum or invades
      other organs

Note: For any T, add (m) for multiple tumours.

N – Regional Lymph Nodes

NX   Regional lymph nodes cannot be assessed
N0   No regional lymph node metastasis
N1   Regional lymph node metastasis

M – Distant Metastasis

M0   No distant metastasis
M1   Distant metastasis

pTNM Pathological Classification

The pT and pN categories correspond to the T and N
categories. For pM see page 15.

G Histopathological Grading

The following grading scheme has been proposed for gastrointestinal carcinoids:

Grade	Mitotic count (per 10 HPF)[1]	Ki-67 index (%)[2]
G1	<2	≤2
G2	2–20	3–20
G3	>20	>20

[1]10 HPF: high power field = 2 mm², at least 40 fields (at 40 × magnification) evaluated in areas of highest mitotic density.

[2]Ki-67/MIB1 antibody: % of 2000 tumour cells in areas of highest nuclear labelling.

Stage Grouping (Non appendiceal GI carcinoids)

Stage I	T1	N0	M0
Stage IIA	T2	N0	M0
Stage IIB	T3	N0	M0
Stage IIIA	T4	N0	M0
Stage IIIB	Any T	N1	M0
Stage IV	Any T	Any N	M1

Summary

Stomach: Carcinoid

Tis	Mucosa <0.5 mm
T1	Mucosa 0.5 mm to 1 cm or submucosa ≤1 cm
T2	Muscularis propria or >1 cm
T3	Subserosa
T4	Perforates serosa; adjacent structures

Small Intestine: Carcinoid

T1	Lamina propria or submucosa and ≤1 cm
T2	Muscularis propria or >1 cm
T3	Jejunal, ileal: subserosa
	Ampullary, duodenal: invades pancreas or retroperitoneum
T4	Perforates serosa; adjacent structures

Large intestine: Carcinoid

T1	Lamina propria or submucosa and ≤2 cm
T1a	<1 cm
T1b	1–2 cm
T2	Muscularis propria or >2 cm
T3	Subserosa, or pericolorectal tissue
T4	Perforates serosa; adjacent structures

Colon and Rectum
(ICD-O C18–20)

Rules for Classification

The classification applies to carcinomas. There should be histological confirmation of the disease.

The following are the procedures for assessing the T, N, and M categories:

T categories	Physical examination, imaging, endoscopy, and/or surgical exploration
N categories	Physical examination, imaging, and/or surgical exploration
M categories	Physical examination, imaging, and/or surgical exploration

Anatomical Sites and Subsites

Colon (C18)
1. Caecum (C18.0)
2. Ascending colon (C18.2)
3. Hepatic flexure (C18.3)
4. Transverse colon (C18.4)
5. Splenic flexure (C18.5)
6. Descending colon (C18.6)
7. Sigmoid colon (C18.7)

Rectosigmoid junction (C19)

Rectum (C20)

Regional Lymph Nodes

For each anatomical site or subsite the following are regional lymph nodes:

Caecum	Ileocolic, right colic
Ascending colon	Ileocolic, right colic, middle colic,
Hepatic flexure	Right colic, middle colic
Transverse colon	Right colic, middle colic, left colic, inferior mesenteric
Splenic flexure	Middle colic, left colic, inferior mesenteric
Descending colon	Left colic, inferior mesenteric
Sigmoid colon	Sigmoid, left colic, superior rectal (haemorrhoidal), inferior mesenteric, rectosigmoid
Rectum	Superior, middle, and inferior rectal (haemorrhoidal), inferior mesenteric, internal iliac, mesorectal (pararectal), lateral sacral, presacral, sacral promontory (Gerota)

Metastasis in nodes other than those listed above is classified as distant metastasis.

TNM Clinical Classification

T – Primary Tumour

TX   Primary tumour cannot be assessed
T0   No evidence of primary tumour
Tis[1]   Carcinoma in situ: intraepithelial or invasion of lamina propria

T1   Tumour invades submucosa
T2   Tumour invades muscularis propria
T3   Tumour invades subserosa or into non-peritonealized pericolic or perirectal tissues
T4   Tumour directly invades other organs or structures and/or perforates visceral peritoneum
    T4a   Tumour perforates visceral peritoneum
    T4b   Tumour directly invades other organs or structures[2,3]

Notes: 1. Tis includes cancer cells confined within the glandular basement membrane (intraepithelial) or mucosal lamina propria (intramucosal) with no extension through the muscularis mucosae into the submucosa.
       2. Direct invasion in T4b includes invasion of other organs or segments of the colorectum by way of the serosa, as confirmed on microscopic examination, or for tumours in a retroperitoneal or subperitoneal location, direct invasion of other organs or structures by virtue of extension beyond the muscularis propria.
       3. Tumour that is adherent to other organs or structures, macroscopically, is classified cT4b. However, if no tumour is present in the adhesion, microscopically, the classification should be pT1–3, depending on the anatomical depth of wall invasion.

N – Regional Lymph Nodes

NX   Regional lymph nodes cannot be assessed
N0   No regional lymph node metastasis

N1   Metastasis in 1–3 regional lymph nodes
      N1a Metastasis in 1 regional lymph node
      N1b Metastasis in 2–3 regional lymph nodes
      N1c Tumour deposit(s), i.e., satellites*, in the
           subserosa, or in non-peritonealized pericolic
           or perirectal soft tissue *without* regional
           lymph node metastasis
N2   Metastasis in 4 or more regional lymph nodes
      N2a Metastasis in 4–6 regional lymph nodes
      N2b Metastasis in 7 or more regional lymph
           nodes

Note: *Tumour deposits (satellites), i.e., macroscopic or microscopic nests or nodules, in the pericolorectal adipose
tissue's lymph drainage area of a primary carcinoma
without histological evidence of residual lymph node
in the nodule, may represent discontinuous spread,
venous invasion with extravascular spread (V1/2) or a
totally replaced lymph node (N1/2). If such deposits are
observed with lesions that would otherwise be classified
as T1 or T2, then the T classification is not changed, but
the nodule(s) is recorded as N1c. If a nodule is considered by the pathologist to be a totally replaced lymph
node (generally having a smooth contour), it should be
recorded as a positive lymph node and not as a satellite, and each nodule should be counted separately as a
lymph node in the final pN determination.

M – Distant Metastasis

M0   No distant metastasis
M1   Distant metastasis
      M1a Metastasis confined to one organ (liver,
           lung, ovary, non-regional lymph node(s))
      M1b Metastasis in more than one organ or the
           peritoneum

TNM Pathological Classification

The pT and pN categories correspond to the T and N categories. For pM see page 15.

pN0   Histological examination of a regional lymphadenectomy specimen will ordinarily include 12 or more lymph nodes.

If the lymph nodes are negative, but the number ordinarily examined is not met, classify as pN0.

G Histopathological Grading

See definitions on page 65.

Stage Grouping

Stage 0	Tis	N0	M0
Stage I	T1, T2	N0	M0
Stage II	T3, T4	N0	M0
Stage IIA	T3	N0	M0
Stage IIB	T4a	N0	M0
Stage IIC	T4b	N0	M0
Stage III	Any T	N1, N2	M0
Stage IIIA	T1, T2	N1	M0
	T1	N2a	M0
Stage IIIB	T3, T4a	N1	M0
	T2, T3	N2a	M0
	T1, T2	N2b	M0
Stage IIIC	T4a	N2a	M0
	T3, T4a	N2b	M0
	T4b	N1, N2	M0
Stage IVA	Any T	Any N	M1a
Stage IVB	Any T	Any N	M1b

Summary

Colon and Rectum	
T1	Submucosa
T2	Muscularis propria
T3	Subserosa, pericolorectal tissues
T4a	Visceral peritoneum
T4b	Other organs or structures
N1a	1 regional
N1b	2–3 regional
N1c	Satellite(s) without regional nodes
N2a	4–6 regional
N2b	7 or more regional
M1a	1 organ
M1b	>1 organ, peritoneum

Anal Canal
(ICD-O C21.1)

The anal canal extends from rectum to perianal skin (to the junction with hair-bearing skin). It is lined by the mucous membrane overlying the internal sphincter, including the transitional epithelium and dentate line. Tumours of anal margin (ICD-O C44.5) are classified with skin tumours (page 165).

Rules for Classification

The classification applies to carcinomas. There should be histological confirmation of the disease and division of cases by histological type.

The following are the procedures for assessing T, N, and M categories:

T categories	Physical examination, imaging, endoscopy, and/or surgical exploration
N categories	Physical examination, imaging, and/or surgical exploration
M categories	Physical examination, imaging, and/or surgical exploration

Regional Lymph Nodes

The regional lymph nodes are the perirectal, the internal iliac, and the inguinal lymph nodes.

TNM Clinical Classification

T – Primary Tumour

TX	Primary tumour cannot be assessed
T0	No evidence of primary tumour
Tis	Carcinoma in situ, Bowen disease, High-grade Squamous Intraepithelial Lesion (HSIL), Anal Intraepithelial Neoplasia II–III (AIN II–III)

T1	Tumour 2 cm or less in greatest dimension
T2	Tumour more than 2 cm but not more than 5 cm in greatest dimension
T3	Tumour more than 5 cm in greatest dimension
T4	Tumour of any size invades adjacent organ(s), e.g., vagina, urethra, bladder[1]

Note: 1. Direct invasion of the rectal wall, perianal skin, subcutaneous tissue, or the sphincter muscle(s) *alone* is not classified as T4.

N – Regional Lymph Nodes

NX	Regional lymph nodes cannot be assessed
N0	No regional lymph node metastasis
N1	Metastasis in perirectal lymph node(s)
N2	Metastasis in unilateral internal iliac and/or unilateral inguinal lymph node(s)
N3	Metastasis in perirectal and inguinal lymph nodes and/or bilateral internal iliac and/or bilateral inguinal lymph nodes

M – Distant Metastasis

M0	No distant metastasis
M1	Distant metastasis

pTNM Pathological Classification

The pT and pN categories correspond to the T and N categories. For pM see page 15.

pN0   Histological examination of a regional per-irectal/pelvic lymphadenectomy specimen will ordinarily include 12 or more lymph nodes; histological examination of an inguinal lymphadenectomy specimen will ordinarily include 6 or more lymph nodes.

If the lymph nodes are negative, but the number ordinarily examined is not met, classify as pN0.

G Histopathological Grading

See definitions on page 65.

Stage Grouping

Stage 0	Tis	N0	M0
Stage I	T1	N0	M0
Stage II	T2, T3	N0	M0
Stage IIIA	T1, T2, T3	N1	M0
	T4	N0	M0
Stage IIIB	T4	N1	M0
	Any T	N2, N3	M0
Stage IV	Any T	Any N	M1

Summary

Anal Canal	
T1	≤2 cm
T2	>2 cm to 5 cm
T3	>5 cm
T4	Adjacent organ(s)
N1	Perirectal
N2	Unilateral internal iliac/inguinal
N3	Perirectal and inguinal, bilateral internal iliac/inguinal

Liver - Hepatocellular Carcinoma
(ICD-O C22.0)

Rules for Classification

The classification applies to hepatocellular carcinoma.

Cholangio- (intrahepatic bile duct) carcinoma of the liver has a separate classification (see page 114). There should be histological confirmation of the disease.

The following are the procedures for assessing T, N, and M categories:

T categories	Physical examination, imaging, and/or surgical exploration
N categories	Physical examination, imaging, and/or surgical exploration
M categories	Physical examination, imaging, and/or surgical exploration

Note: Although the presence of cirrhosis is an important prognostic factor it does not affect the TNM classification, being an independent prognostic variable.

Regional Lymph Nodes

The regional lymph nodes are the hilar, hepatic (along the proper hepatic artery), periportal (along the portal vein) and those along the abdominal inferior vena cava above the renal veins (except the inferior phrenic nodes).

TNM Clinical Classification

T – Primary Tumour

TX   Primary tumour cannot be assessed
T0   No evidence of primary tumour

T1   Solitary tumour without vascular invasion
T2   Solitary tumour with vascular invasion *or* multiple tumours, none more than 5 cm in greatest dimension
T3   Multiple tumours any more than 5 cm *or* tumour involving a major branch of the portal or hepatic vein(s)

      T3a   Multiple tumours any more than 5 cm
      T3b   Tumour involving a major branch of the portal or hepatic vein(s)

T4   Tumour(s) with direct invasion of adjacent organs other than the gallbladder *or* with perforation of visceral peritoneum

N – Regional Lymph Nodes

NX   Regional lymph nodes cannot be assessed
N0   No regional lymph node metastasis
N1   Regional lymph node metastasis

M – Distant Metastasis

M0   No distant metastasis
M1   Distant metastasis

pTNM Pathological Classification

The pT and pN categories correspond to the T and N categories. For pM see page 15.

pN0   Histological examination of a regional lymphadenectomy specimen will ordinarily include 3 or more lymph nodes.

If the lymph nodes are negative, but the number ordinarily examined is not met, classify as pN0.

G Histopathological Grading

For histopathological grading see: Edmondson HA, Steiner PE. Primary carcinoma of the liver: a study of 100 cases among 48,900 necropsies. *Cancer* 1954; 7:462–504.

Edmonson/Steiner grades are numbered Grades 1, 2, 3, and 4.

Stage Grouping

Liver

Stage			
Stage I	T1	N0	M0
Stage II	T2	N0	M0
Stage IIIA	T3a	N0	M0
Stage IIIB	T3b	N0	M0
Stage IIIC	T4	N0	M0
Stage IVA	Any T	N1	M0
Stage IVB	Any T	Any N	M1

Summary

Liver - Hepatocellular carcinoma

T1	Solitary without vascular invasion
T2	Solitary with vascular invasion, multiple ≤5 cm
T3	(a) Multiple >5 cm
	(b) Invades major branch of portal or hepatic vein
T4	Invades adjacent organs other than gallbladder
	Perforates visceral peritoneum
N1	Regional

Liver - Intrahepatic Bile Ducts
(ICD-O C22.1)

Rules for Classification

The staging system applies to intrahepatic cholangiocarcinoma, cholangiocellular carcinoma, and combined hepatocellular and cholangiocarcinoma (mixed hepatocellular/cholangiocellular carcinoma).

The following are the procedures for assessing T, N, and M categories:

T categories	Physical examination, imaging, and/or surgical exploration
N categories	Physical examination, imaging, and/or surgical exploration
M categories	Physical examination, imaging, and/or surgical exploration

Regional Lymph Nodes

For right-liver intrahepatic cholangiocarcinoma, the regional lymph nodes include the hilar (common bile duct, hepatic arteries, portal vein, and cystic duct), periduodenal and peripancreatic lymph nodes.

For left-liver intrahepatic cholangiocarcinoma, regional lymph nodes include hilar and gastrohepatic lymph nodes.

For intrahepatic cholangiocarcinoma, spread to the coeliac and/or periaortic and caval lymph nodes is distant metastasis (M1).

TNM Clinical Classification

T – Primary Tumour

TX   Primary tumour cannot be assessed
T0   No evidence of primary tumour
Tis   Carcinoma in situ (intraductal tumour)

T1   Solitary tumour without vascular invasion
T2a   Solitary tumour with vascular invasion
T2b   Multiple tumours, with or without vascular invasion
T3   Tumour perforates the visceral peritoneum or directly invades adjacent extrahepatic structures
T4   Tumour with periductal invasion (periductal growth pattern)

N – Regional Lymph Nodes

NX   Regional lymph nodes cannot be assessed
N0   No regional lymph node metastasis
N1   Regional lymph node metastasis

M – Distant Metastasis

M0   No distant metastasis
M1   Distant metastasis

pTNM Pathological Classification

The pT and pN categories correspond to the T and N categories. For pM see page 15.

pN0 Histological examination of a regional lymphadenectomy specimen will ordinarily include 3 or more lymph nodes.

If the regional lymph nodes are negative, but the number ordinarily examined is not met, classify as pN0.

G Histopathological Grading

See definitions on page 65.

Stage Grouping

Stage I	T1	N0	M0
Stage II	T2	N0	M0
Stage III	T3	N0	M0
Stage IVA	T4	N0	M0
	Any T	N1	M0
Stage IVB	Any T	Any N	M1

Summary

Intrahepatic bile ducts
T1   Solitary without vascular invasion
T2a   Solitary with vascular invasion
T2b   Multiple
T3   Perforates visceral peritoneum or invades adjacent extrahepatic structures
T4   Periductal invasion
N1   Regional

Gallbladder
(ICD-O C23)

Rules for Classification

The classification applies to carcinomas of gall-bladder and cystic duct. There should be histological confirmation of the disease.

The following are the procedures for assessing T, N, and M categories:

T categories	Physical examination, imaging, and/or surgical exploration
N categories	Physical examination, imaging, and/or surgical exploration
M categories	Physical examination, imaging, and/or surgical exploration

Regional Lymph Nodes

Regional lymph nodes are the hepatic hilus nodes (including nodes along the common bile duct, common hepatic artery, portal vein, and cystic duct).

Coeliac, periduodenal, peripancreatic, and superior mesenteric artery node involvement is considered distant metastasis (M1).

TNM Clinical Classification

T – Primary Tumour

TX   Primary tumour cannot be assessed
T0   No evidence of primary tumour
Tis   Carcinoma in situ

T1   Tumour invades lamina propria or muscular layer
      T1a Tumour invades lamina propria
      T1b Tumour invades muscular layer
T2   Tumour invades perimuscular connective tissue; no extension beyond serosa or into liver
T3   Tumour perforates the serosa (visceral peritoneum) and/or directly invades the liver and/or one other adjacent organ or structure, such as stomach, duodenum, colon, pancreas, omentum, extrahepatic bile ducts
T4   Tumour invades main portal vein or hepatic artery or invades two or more extrahepatic organs or structures

N – Regional Lymph Nodes

NX   Regional lymph nodes cannot be assessed
N0   No regional lymph node metastasis
N1   Regional lymph node metastasis (including nodes along the cystic duct, common bile duct, common hepatic artery, and portal vein).

M – Distant Metastasis

M0 No distant metastasis
M1 Distant metastasis

pTNM Pathological Classification

The pT and pN categories correspond to the T and N categories. For pM see page 15.

pN0 Histological examination of a regional lymphadenectomy specimen will ordinarily include 3 or more lymph nodes.
If the regional lymph nodes are negative, but the number ordinarily examined is not met, classify as pN0.

G Histopathological Grading

See definitions on page 65.

Stage Grouping

Stage 0	Tis	N0	M0
Stage I	T1	N0	M0
Stage II	T2	N0	M0
Stage IIIA	T3	N0	M0
Stage IIIB	T1, T2, T3	N1	M0
Stage IVA	T4	Any N	M0
Stage IVB	Any T	Any N	M1

Summary

Gallbladder	
T1	Lamina propria or muscular layer
	T1a Lamina propria
	T1b Muscular layer
T2	Perimuscular connective tissue
T3	Serosa, one organ, and/or liver
T4	Portal vein, hepatic artery, or two or more extrahepatic organs
N1	Along cystic duct, common bile duct, common hepatic artery, portal vein

Extrahepatic Bile Ducts - Perihilar
(ICD-O C24.0)

Rules for Classification

The classification applies to carcinomas of the extrahepatic bile ducts of perihilar localization (Klatskin tumour). Included are the right, left, and the common hepatic ducts.

The following are the procedures for assessing T, N, and M categories:

T categories	Physical examination, imaging, and/or surgical exploration
N categories	Physical examination, imaging, and/or surgical exploration
M categories	Physical examination, imaging, and/or surgical exploration

Anatomical Sites and Subsites

Perihilar cholangiocarcinomas are tumours located in the extrahepatic biliary tree proximal to the origin of the cystic duct.

Regional Lymph Nodes

The regional nodes are the hilar and pericholedochal nodes in the hepatoduodenal ligament.

TNM Clinical Classification

T – Primary Tumour

TX Primary tumour cannot be assessed
T0 No evidence of primary tumour
Tis Carcinoma in situ

T1 Tumour confined to the bile duct, with extension up to the muscle layer or fibrous tissue
T2a Tumour invades beyond the wall of the bile duct to surrounding adipose tissue
T2b Tumour invades adjacent hepatic parenchyma
T3 Tumour invades unilateral branches of the portal vein or hepatic artery
T4 Tumour invades the main portal vein or its branches bilaterally; or the common hepatic artery; or the second-order biliary radicals bilaterally; or unilateral second-order biliary radicals with contralateral portal vein or hepatic artery involvement

N – Regional Lymph Nodes

NX Regional lymph nodes cannot be assessed
N0 No regional lymph node metastasis
N1 Regional lymph node metastasis including nodes along the cystic duct, common bile duct, common hepatic artery, and portal vein

M – Distant Metastasis

M0 No distant metastasis
M1 Distant metastasis

pTNM Pathological Classification

The pT and pN categories correspond to the T and N categories. For pM see page 15.

pN0   Histological examination of a regional lymphadenectomy specimen will ordinarily include 15 or more lymph nodes.

If the regional lymph nodes are negative, but the number ordinarily examined is not met, classify as pN0.

G Histopathological Grading

See definitions on page 65.

Stage Grouping

Stage 0	Tis	N0	M0
Stage I	T1	N0	M0
Stage II	T2a, T2b	N0	M0
Stage IIIA	T3	N0	M0
Stage IIIB	T1, T2, T3	N1	M0
Stage IVA	T4	N0, N1	M0
Stage IVB	Any T	Any N	M1

Summary

Perihilar bile ducts

T1	Ductal wall
T2a	Beyond ductal wall
T2b	Adjacent hepatic parenchyma
T3	Unilateral branches of portal vein or hepatic artery
T4	Main portal vein; bilateral branches; common hepatic artery; second-order biliary radicals bilaterally; unilateral second-order biliary radicals with contralateral portal vein or hepatic artery involvement
N1	Nodes along cystic duct, common bile duct, common hepatic artery, portal vein

Extrahepatic Bile Ducts - Distal
(ICD-O C24.0)

Rules for Classification

The classification applies to carcinomas of the extrahepatic bile ducts distal to the insertion of the cystic duct. Cystic duct carcinoma is included under gallbladder.

The following are the procedures for assessing T, N, and M categories:

T categories	Physical examination, imaging, and/or surgical exploration
N categories	Physical examination, imaging, and/or surgical exploration
M categories	Physical examination, imaging, and/or surgical exploration

Regional Lymph Nodes

The regional lymph nodes are along the common bile duct, common hepatic artery, back towards the coeliac trunk, posterior and anterior pancreaticoduodenal nodes, and nodes along the superior mesenteric vein and the right lateral wall of the superior mesenteric artery.

TNM Clinical Classification

T – Primary Tumour

TX   Primary tumour cannot be assessed
T0   No evidence of primary tumour
Tis   Carcinoma in situ

T1   Tumour confined to the bile duct
T2   Tumour invades beyond the wall of the bile duct
T3   Tumour invades the gallbladder, liver, pancreas, duodenum, or other adjacent organs
T4   Tumour involves the coeliac axis or the superior mesenteric artery

N – Regional Lymph Nodes

NX   Regional lymph nodes cannot be assessed
N0   No regional lymph node metastasis
N1   Regional lymph node metastasis

M – Distant Metastasis

M0   No distant metastasis
M1   Distant metastasis

pTNM Pathological Classification

The pT and pN categories correspond to the T and N categories. For pM see page 15.

pN0   Histological examination of a regional lymphadenectomy specimen will ordinarily include 12 or more lymph nodes.

    If the regional lymph nodes are negative, but the number ordinarily examined is not met, classify as pN0.

G Histopathological Grading

See definitions on page 65.

Stage Grouping

Stage 0	Tis	N0	M0
Stage IA	T1	N0	M0
Stage IB	T2	N0	M0
Stage IIA	T3	N0	M0
Stage IIB	T1, T2, T3	N1	M0
Stage III	T4	Any N	M0
Stage IV	Any T	Any N	M1

Summary

Distal Extrahepatic Bile Ducts	
T1	Ductal wall
T2	Beyond ductal wall
T3	Gallbladder, pancreas, duodenum, adjacent organs
T4	Coeliac axis or superior mesenteric artery
N1	Regional

Ampulla of Vater
(ICD-O C24.1)

Rules for Classification

The classification applies only to carcinomas. There should be histological confirmation of the disease.

The following are the procedures for assessing T, N, and M categories:

T categories	Physical examination, imaging, and/or surgical exploration
N categories	Physical examination, imaging, and/or surgical exploration
M categories	Physical examination, imaging, and/or surgical exploration

Regional Lymph Nodes

The regional lymph nodes are:

Superior	Superior to head and body of pancreas
Inferior	Inferior to head and body of pancreas
Anterior	Anterior pancreaticoduodenal, pyloric, and proximal mesenteric
Posterior	Posterior pancreaticoduodenal, common bile duct, and proximal mesenteric

Note: The splenic lymph nodes and those of the tail of the pancreas are *not* regional; metastases to these lymph nodes are coded M1.

TNM Clinical Classification

T – Primary Tumour

TX   Primary tumour cannot be assessed
T0   No evidence of primary tumour
Tis   Carcinoma in situ

T1   Tumour limited to ampulla of Vater or sphincter of Oddi
T2   Tumour invades duodenal wall
T3   Tumour invades pancreas
T4   Tumour invades peripancreatic soft tissues, or other adjacent organs or structures

N – Regional Lymph Nodes

NX   Regional lymph nodes cannot be assessed
N0   No regional lymph node metastasis
N1   Regional lymph node metastasis

M – Distant Metastasis

M0   No distant metastasis
M1   Distant metastasis

pTNM Pathological Classification

The pT and pN categories correspond to the T and N categories. For pM see page 65.

pN0   Histological examination of a regional lymphadenectomy specimen will ordinarily include 10 or more lymph nodes.

If the lymph nodes are negative, but the number ordinarily examined is not met, classify as pN0.

G Histopathological Grading

See definitions on page 65.

Stage Grouping

Stage 0	Tis	N0	M0
Stage IA	T1	N0	M0
Stage IB	T2	N0	M0
Stage IIA	T3	N0	M0
Stage IIB	T1, T2, T3	N1	M0
Stage III	T4	Any N	M0
Stage IV	Any T	Any N	M1

Summary

Ampulla of Vater	
T1	Ampulla or sphincter of Oddi
T2	Duodenal wall
T3	Pancreas
T4	Beyond pancreas
N1	Regional

Pancreas
(ICD-O C25)

Rules for Classification

The classification applies to carcinomas of the exocrine pancreas and pancreatic neuroendocrine tumours including carcinoids. There should be histological or cytological confirmation of the disease.

The following are the procedures for assessing T, N, and M categories:

T categories	Physical examination, imaging, and/or surgical exploration
N categories	Physical examination, imaging, and/or surgical exploration
M categories	Physical examination, imaging, and/or surgical exploration

Anatomical Subsites

C25.0   Head of pancreas[1]
C25.1   Body of pancreas[2]
C25.2   Tail of pancreas[3]
C25.3   Pancreatic duct
C25.4   Islets of Langerhans (endocrine pancreas)

Notes: 1. Tumours of the head of the pancreas are those arising to the right of the left border of the superior mesenteric vein. The uncinate process is considered as part of the head.

2. Tumours of the body are those arising between the left border of the superior mesenteric vein and left border of the aorta.
3. Tumours of the tail are those arising between the left border of the aorta and the hilum of the spleen.

Regional Lymph Nodes

The regional lymph nodes are the peripancreatic nodes, which may be subdivided as follows:

Superior	Superior to head and body
Inferior	Inferior to head and body
Anterior	Anterior pancreaticoduodenal, pyloric (for tumours of head only), and proximal mesenteric
Posterior	Posterior pancreaticoduodenal, common bile duct, and proximal mesenteric
Splenic	Hilum of spleen and tail of pancreas (for tumours of body and tail only)
Coeliac	(for tumours of head only)

TNM Clinical Classification

T – Primary Tumour

TX   Primary tumour cannot be assessed
T0   No evidence of primary tumour
Tis Carcinoma in situ*

T1   Tumour limited to pancreas, 2 cm or less in greatest dimension
T2   Tumour limited to pancreas, more than 2 cm in greatest dimension

T3   Tumour extends beyond pancreas, but with-
      out involvement of coeliac axis or superior
      mesenteric artery
T4   Tumour involves coeliac axis or superior
      mesenteric artery

■ **Note:**   *Tis also includes the 'PanIN–III' classification.

N – Regional Lymph Nodes

NX   Regional lymph nodes cannot be assessed
N0   No regional lymph node metastasis
N1   Regional lymph node metastasis

M – Distant Metastasis

M0   No distant metastasis
M1   Distant metastasis

pTNM Pathological Classification

The pT and pN categories correspond to the T and N
categories. For pM see page 15.

pN0   Histological examination of a regional lym-
          phadenectomy specimen will ordinarily include
          10 or more lymph nodes.

          If the lymph nodes are negative, but the
          number ordinarily examined is not met, classify
          as pN0.

G Histopathological Grading

See definitions on page 65.

Stage Grouping

Stage 0	Tis	N0	M0
Stage IA	T1	N0	M0
Stage IB	T2	N0	M0
Stage IIA	T3	N0	M0
Stage IIB	T1, T2, T3	N1	M0
Stage III	T4	Any N	M0
Stage IV	Any T	Any N	M1

Summary

Pancreas	
T1	Limited to pancreas ≤2 cm
T2	Limited to pancreas >2 cm
T3	Beyond pancreas
T4	Coeliac axis or superior mesenteric artery
N1	Regional

LUNG AND PLEURAL TUMOURS

Introductory Notes

The classifications apply to carcinomas of the lung including non-small cell and small cell carcinomas, bronchopulmonary carcinoid tumours, and malignant mesothelioma of pleura.

Each site is described under the following headings:

- Rules for classification with the procedures for assessing T, N, and M categories; additional methods may be used when they enhance the accuracy of appraisal before treatment
- Anatomical subsites where appropriate
- Definition of the regional lymph nodes
- TNM Clinical classification
- pTNM Pathological classification
- G Histopathological grading where applicable
- Stage grouping
- Summary

Regional Lymph Nodes

The regional lymph nodes extend from the supraclavicular region to the diaphragm. Direct extension of the primary tumour into lymph nodes is classified as lymph node metastasis.

Distant Metastasis

The categories M1 and pM1 may be further specified according to the following notation:

Pulmonary	PUL	Bone marrow	MAR
Osseous	OSS	Pleura	PLE
Hepatic	HEP	Peritoneum	PER
Brain	BRA	Adrenals	ADR
Lymph nodes	LYM	Skin	SKI
Others	OTH		

R Classification

See Introduction, page 19.

Lung
(ICD-O C34)

Rules for Classification

The classification applies to carcinomas of the lung including non-small cell carcinomas, small cell carcinomas, and bronchopulmonary carcinoid tumours. It does not apply to sarcomas and other rare tumours.

Changes to the sixth edition are based upon recommendations from the International Association for the Study of Lung Cancer (IASLC) Staging Project (see references below).

There should be histological confirmation of the disease and division of cases by histological type.

The following are the procedures for assessing T, N, and M categories:

T categories	Physical examination, imaging, endoscopy, and/or surgical exploration
N categories	Physical examination, imaging, endoscopy, and/or surgical exploration
M categories	Physical examination, imaging, and/or surgical exploration

Anatomical Subsites

1. Main bronchus (C34.0)
2. Upper lobe (C34.1)
3. Middle lobe (C34.2)
4. Lower lobe (C34.3)

Regional Lymph Nodes

The regional lymph nodes are the intrathoracic nodes (mediastinal, hilar, lobar, interlobar, segmental, and subsegmental), scalene, and supraclavicular lymph nodes.

TNM Clinical Classification

T – Primary Tumour

TX Primary tumour cannot be assessed, *or* tumour proven by the presence of malignant cells in sputum or bronchial washings but not visualized by imaging or bronchoscopy

T0 No evidence of primary tumour

Tis Carcinoma in situ

T1 Tumour 3 cm or less in greatest dimension, surrounded by lung or visceral pleura, without bronchoscopic evidence of invasion more proximal than the lobar bronchus (i.e., not in the main bronchus)[1]

   T1a Tumour 2 cm or less in greatest dimension[1]

   T1b Tumour more than 2 cm but not more than 3 cm in greatest dimension[1]

T2   Tumour more than 3 cm but not more than 7 cm; or tumour with *any* of the following features[2]
- Involves main bronchus, 2 cm or more distal to the carina
- Invades visceral pleura
- Associated with atelectasis or obstructive pneumonitis that extends to the hilar region but does not involve the entire lung

    T2a   Tumour more than 3 cm but not more than 5 cm in greatest dimension

    T2b   Tumour more than 5 cm but not more than 7 cm in greatest dimension

T3   Tumour more than 7 cm or one that directly invades any of the following: chest wall (including superior sulcus tumours), diaphragm, phrenic nerve, mediastinal pleura, parietal pericardium; *or* tumour in the main bronchus less than 2 cm distal to the carina[1] but without involvement of the carina; *or* associated atelectasis or obstructive pneumonitis of the entire lung or separate tumour nodule(s) in the same lobe as the primary

T4   Tumour of any size that invades any of the following: mediastinum, heart, great vessels, trachea, recurrent laryngeal nerve, oesophagus, vertebral body, carina; separate tumour nodule(s) in a different ipsilateral lobe to that of the primary

N – Regional Lymph Nodes

NX   Regional lymph nodes cannot be assessed

N0   No regional lymph node metastasis

N1   Metastasis in ipsilateral peribronchial and/or ipsilateral hilar lymph nodes and intrapulmonary nodes, including involvement by direct extension

N2   Metastasis in ipsilateral mediastinal and/or subcarinal lymph node(s)

N3   Metastasis in contralateral mediastinal, contralateral hilar, ipsilateral or contralateral scalene, or supraclavicular lymph node(s)

M – Distant Metastasis

M0   No distant metastasis
M1   Distant metastasis
    M1a Separate tumour nodule(s) in a contralateral lobe; tumour with pleural nodules or malignant pleural or pericardial effusion[3]
    M1b Distant metastasis

Notes: 1. The uncommon superficial spreading tumour of any size with its invasive component limited to the bronchial wall, which may extend proximal to the main bronchus, is also classified as T1a.

2. T2 tumours with these features are classified T2a if 5 cm or less, or if size cannot be determined and T2b if greater than 5 cm but not larger than 7 cm.

3. Most pleural (pericardial) effusions with lung cancer are due to tumour. In a few patients, however, multiple microscopical examinations of pleural (pericardial) fluid are negative for tumour, and the fluid is non-bloody and is not an exudate. Where these elements and clinical judgement dictate that the effusion is not related to the tumour, the effusion should be excluded as a staging element and the patient should be classified as M0.

pTNM Pathological Classification

The pT and pN categories correspond to the T and N categories. For pM see page 15.

pN0 Histological examination of hilar and mediastinal lymphadenectomy specimen(s) will ordinarily include 6 or more lymph nodes/stations. Three of these nodes/stations should be mediastinal, including the subcarinal nodes and 3 from N1 nodes/stations. Labelling according to the IASLC chart and table of definitions given in the TNM Supplement is desirable. If all the lymph nodes examined are negative, but the number ordinarily examined is not met, classify as pN0.

G Histopathological Grading

GX   Grade of differentiation cannot be assessed
G1   Well differentiated
G2   Moderately differentiated
G3   Poorly differentiated
G4   Undifferentiated

Stage Grouping

Occult carcinoma	TX	N0	M0
Stage 0	Tis	N0	M0
Stage IA	T1a, b	N0	M0
Stage IB	T2a	N0	M0
Stage IIA	T2b	N0	M0
	T1a, b	N1	M0
	T2a	N1	M0
Stage IIB	T2b	N1	M0
	T3	N0	M0
Stage IIIA	T1a, b, T2a, b	N2	M0
	T3	N1, N2	M0
	T4	N0, N1	M0
Stage IIIB	T4	N2	M0
	Any T	N3	M0
Stage IV	Any T	Any N	M1

Summary

Lung	
TX	Positive cytology only
T1	≤3 cm
T1a	≤2 cm
T1b	>2–3 cm
T2	Main bronchus ≥2 cm from carina, invades visceral pleura, partial atelectasis
T2a	>3 cm to 5 cm
T2b	>5 cm to 7 cm
T3	>7 cm; chest wall, diaphragm, pericardium, mediastinal pleura, main bronchus <2 cm from carina, total atelectasis, separate nodule(s) in same lobe
T4	Mediastinum, heart, great vessels, carina, trachea, oesophagus, vertebral body; separate tumour nodule(s) in a different ipsilateral lobe
N1	Ipsilateral peribronchial, ipsilateral hilar
N2	Ipsilateral mediastinal, subcarinal
N3	Contralateral mediastinal or hilar, scalene or supraclavicular
M1	Distant metastasis
M1a	Separate tumour nodule(s) in a contralateral lobe; pleural nodules or malignant pleural or pericardial effusion
M1b	Distant metastasis

References

Goldstraw P, Crowley J et al. THE IASLC International staging project on lung cancer. *J Thor Oncol* 2006; 1:281–286.

Goldstraw P, Crowley J, Chansky K, et al. on behalf of the International Staging Committee. The IASLC Lung Cancer Staging Project: Proposals for the revision of the TNM stage groupings in the forthcoming (seventh) edition of the *TNM Classification of Malignant Tumours. J Thor Oncol* 2007; 2:706–714.

Groome PA, Bolejack V, Crowley J, et al. on behalf of the International Staging Committee. The IASLC Lung Cancer Staging Project: Validation of the proposals for revision of the T, N, and M descriptors and consequent stage groupings in the forthcoming (seventh) edition of the *TNM Classification of Malignant Tumours. J Thor Oncol* 2007; 2:694–705.

Postmus PE, Brambilla E, Chansky K, et al. on behalf of the IASLC Staging Committee. The IASLC Lung Cancer Staging Project: Proposals for the Revision of the M descriptors in the forthcoming (seventh) edition of the *TNM Classification for Lung Cancer. J Thor Oncol* 2007; 2:686–693.

Rami-Porta R, Ball D, Crowley J, et al. on behalf of the International Staging Committee. The IASLC Lung Cancer Staging Project: Proposals for the revision of the T descriptors in the forthcoming (seventh) edition of the *TNM Classification of Lung Cancer. J Thor Oncol* 2007; 2:593–602.

Rusch VR, Crowley J, Giroux DJ, et al. on behalf of the International Staging Committee. The IASLC Lung Cancer Staging Project: Proposals for the Revision of the N descriptors in the forthcoming (seventh) edition of the *TNM Classification for Lung Cancer*. *J Thor Oncol* 2007; 2:603–612.

Shepherd FA, Crowley J, van Houtte P, et al. on behalf of the International Staging Committee. The IASLC Lung Cancer Staging Project: Proposals regarding the clinical staging of small cell lung cancer in the forthcoming (seventh) edition of the *TNM Classification of Malignant Tumours*. *J Thor Oncol* 2007; 2:1067–1077.

Travis WD, Giroux DJ, Chansky K, et al. on behalf of the International Staging Committee and Participating Institutions. The IASLC Lung Cancer Staging Project: Proposals for the inclusion of broncho-pulmonary carcinoid tumors in the forthcoming (seventh) edition of the *TNM Classification for Lung Cancer*. *J Thor Oncol* 2008; 3:1213–1223.

Pleural Mesothelioma
(ICD-O C38.4)

Rules for Classification

The classification applies to malignant mesothelioma of the pleura. There should be histological confirmation of the disease.

The following are the procedures for assessing T, N, and M categories:

T categories	Physical examination, imaging, endoscopy, and/or surgical exploration
N categories	Physical examination, imaging, endoscopy, and/or surgical exploration
M categories	Physical examination, imaging, and/or surgical exploration

Regional Lymph Nodes

The regional lymph nodes are the intrathoracic, internal mammary, scalene, and supraclavicular nodes.

TNM Clinical Classification

T – Primary Tumour

TX	Primary tumour cannot be assessed
T0	No evidence of primary tumour

T1   Tumour involves ipsilateral parietal pleura, with or without focal involvement of visceral pleura

   T1a   Tumour involves ipsilateral parietal (mediastinal, diaphragmatic) pleura. No involvement of visceral pleura.

   T1b   Tumour involves ipsilateral parietal (mediastinal, diaphragmatic) pleura, *with* focal involvement of the visceral pleura

T2   Tumour involves any of the ipsilateral pleural surfaces, with at least one the following:
   - Confluent visceral pleura tumour (including the fissure)
   - Invasion of diaphragmatic muscle
   - Invasion of lung parenchyma

T3[1]   Tumour involves any ipsilateral pleural surfaces, with at least one of the following:
   - Invasion of endothoracic fascia
   - Invasion into mediastinal fat
   - Solitary focus of tumour invading soft tissues of the chest wall
   - Non-transmural involvement of the pericardium

T4[2]   Tumour involves any ipsilateral pleural surfaces, with at least one of the following:
   - Diffuse or multifocal invasion of soft tissues of chest wall
   - Any involvement of rib
   - Invasion through diaphragm to peritoneum
   - Invasion of any mediastinal organ(s)
   - Direct extension to contralateral pleura
   - Invasion into the spine

- Extension to internal surface of pericardium
- Pericardial effusion with positive cytology
- Invasion of myocardium
- Invasion of brachial plexus

Notes: 1. T3 describes locally advanced, but potentially resectable tumour.
2. T4 describes locally advanced, technically unresectable tumour.

N – Regional Lymph Nodes

NX   Regional lymph nodes cannot be assessed

N0   No regional lymph node metastasis

N1   Metastasis in ipsilateral bronchopulmonary and/or hilar lymph node(s)

N2   Metastasis in subcarinal lymph node(s) and/or ipsilateral internal mammary or mediastinal lymph node(s)

N3   Metastasis in contralateral mediastinal, internal mammary, or hilar node(s) and/or ipsilateral or contralateral supraclavicular or scalene lymph node(s)

M – Distant Metastasis

M0   No distant metastasis

M1   Distant metastasis

pTNM Pathological Classification

The pT and pN categories correspond to the T and N categories. For pM see page 15.

Stage Grouping

Stage IA	T1a	N0	M0
Stage IB	T1b	N0	M0
Stage II	T2	N0	M0
Stage III	T1, T2	N1	M0
	T1, T2	N2	M0
	T3	N0, N1, N2	M0
Stage IV	T4	Any N	M0
	Any T	N3	M0
	Any T	Any N	M1

Summary

Pleural Mesothelioma

T1	Ipsilateral parietal pleura
T1a	No visceral pleura
T1b	Visceral pleura
T2	Ipsilateral lung, diaphragm, confluent involvement of visceral pleura
T3	Endothoracic fascia, mediastinal fat, focal chest wall, non-transmural pericardium
T4	Contralateral pleura, peritoneum, rib, extensive chest wall or mediastinal invasion, myocardium, brachial plexus, spine, transmural pericardium, malignant pericardial effusion
N1	Ipsilateral bronchopulmonary, hilar
N2	Subcarinal, ipsilateral mediastinal, internal mammary
N3	Contralateral mediastinal, internal mammary, hilar; ipsi/contralateral supraclavicular, scalene

BONE AND SOFT TISSUE TUMOURS

Introductory Notes

The following sites are included:

- Bone
- Soft tissues

Each site is described under the following headings:

- Rules for classification with the procedures for assessing T, N, and M categories; additional methods may be used when they enhance the accuracy of appraisal before treatment
- Anatomical sites where appropriate
- Definition of the regional lymph nodes
- TNM Clinical classification
- pTNM Pathological classification
- G Histopathological grading
- Stage grouping
- Summary

G Histopathological Grading

The staging of bone and soft tissue sarcomas is based on a two-tiered grade classification ('low' vs 'high' grade). Because different grading systems are used, the following is recommended for the translation of three- and four-tiered grading systems into a two-tiered system. In the most commonly employed three-tiered classification, Grade 1 is considered 'low grade' and Grades 2 and 3 'high grade'. In the less common four-tiered systems, Grades 1 and 2 are considered 'low grade' and Grades 3 and 4 'high grade'.

Distant Metastasis

The categories M1 and pM1 may be further specified according to the following notation:

Pulmonary	PUL	Bone marrow	MAR
Osseous	OSS	Pleura	PLE
Hepatic	HEP	Peritoneum	PER
Brain	BRA	Adrenals	ADR
Lymph nodes	LYM	Skin	SKI
Others	OTH		

R Classification

See Introduction, page 19.

Bone
(ICD-O C40, 41)

Rules for Classification

The classification applies to all primary malignant bone tumours except malignant lymphomas, multiple myeloma, surface/juxtacortical osteosarcoma, and juxtacortical chondrosarcoma. There should be histological confirmation of the disease and division of cases by histological type and grade.

The following are the procedures for assessing T, N, and M categories:

T categories	Physical examination and imaging
N categories	Physical examination and imaging
M categories	Physical examination and imaging

Regional Lymph Nodes

The regional lymph nodes are those appropriate to the site of the primary tumour. Regional node involvement is rare and cases in which nodal status is not assessed either clinically or pathologically could be considered N0 instead of NX or pNX.

TNM Clinical Classification

T – Primary Tumour

TX   Primary tumour cannot be assessed
T0   No evidence of primary tumour

T1   Tumour 8 cm or less in greatest dimension
T2   Tumour more than 8 cm in greatest dimension
T3   Discontinuous tumours in the primary bone site

N – Regional Lymph Nodes

NX   Regional lymph nodes cannot be assessed
N0   No regional lymph node metastasis
N1   Regional lymph node metastasis

M – Distant Metastasis

M0   No distant metastasis
M1   Distant metastasis
     M1a   Lung
     M1b   Other distant sites

pTNM Pathological Classification

The pT and pN categories correspond to the T and N categories. For pM see page 15.

G Histopathological Grading

Translation table for three- and four-grade systems to a two-grade (low grade vs high grade) system

TNM two-grade System	Three-grade Systems	Four-grade Systems
Low grade	Grade 1	Grade 1
		Grade 2
High grade	Grade 2	Grade 3
	Grade 3	Grade 4

Note: Ewing sarcoma is classified as high grade. If grade cannot be assessed classify as low grade.

Stage Grouping

Stage IA	T1	N0	M0	Low grade
Stage IB	T2	N0	M0	Low grade
Stage IIA	T1	N0	M0	High grade
Stage IIB	T2	N0	M0	High grade
Stage III	T3	N0	M0	Any grade
Stage IVA	Any T	N0	M1a	Any grade
Stage IVB	Any T	N1	Any M	Any grade
	Any T	Any N	M1b	Any grade

Note: Use N0 for NX

For T1 and T2, use low grade if no grade is stated

Summary

Bone	
T1	≤8 cm
T2	>8 cm
T3	Discontinuous tumours in primary site
N1	Regional
M1a	Lung
M1b	Other sites
	Low grade
	High grade

Soft Tissues
(ICD-O C38.1–3, C47–49)

Rules for Classification

There should be histological confirmation of the disease and division of cases by histological type and grade.

The following are the procedures for assessing T, N, and M categories:

T categories	Physical examination and imaging
N categories	Physical examination and imaging
M categories	Physical examination and imaging

Anatomical Sites

1. Connective, subcutaneous, and other soft tissues (C49), peripheral nerves (C47)
2. Retroperitoneum (C48.0)
3. Mediastinum: anterior (38.1); posterior (C38.2); mediastinum, NOS (C38.3)

Histological Types of Tumour

The following histological types are included, with ICD-O morphology codes:

Alveolar soft part sarcoma	9581/3
Epithelioid sarcoma	8804/3
Extraskeletal chondrosarcoma	9220/3
Extraskeletal osteosarcoma	9180/3
Extraskeletal Ewing sarcoma	9260/3
Primitive neuroectodermal tumour (PNET)	9473/3
Fibrosarcoma	8810/3
Leiomyosarcoma	8890/3
Liposarcoma	8850/3
Malignant fibrous histiocytoma	8830/3
Malignant haemangiopericytoma	9150/3
Malignant mesenchymoma	8990/3
Malignant peripheral nerve sheath tumour	9540/3
Rhabdomyosarcoma	8900/3
Synovial sarcoma	9040/3
Sarcoma, not otherwise specified (NOS)	8800/3

The following histological types are not included:

- Kaposi sarcoma
- Dermatofibrosarcoma (protuberans)
- Fibromatosis (desmoid tumour)
- Sarcoma arising from the dura mater, brain, hollow viscera, or parenchymatous organs (with the exception of breast sarcomas).
- Angiosarcoma, an aggressive sarcoma, is excluded because its natural history is not consistent with the classification.
- Gastrointestinal stromal tumours are separately classified in the Digestive System Tumours section. (See page 78)

Regional Lymph Nodes

The regional lymph nodes are those appropriate to the site of the primary tumour. Regional node involvement is rare and cases in which nodal status is not assessed either clinically or pathologically could be considered N0 instead of NX or pNX.

TNM Clinical Classification

T – Primary Tumour

TX   Primary tumour cannot be assessed
T0   No evidence of primary tumour

T1   Tumour 5 cm or less in greatest dimension
    T1a   Superficial tumour*
    T1b   Deep tumour*
T2   Tumour more than 5 cm in greatest dimension
    T2a   Superficial tumour*
    T2b   Deep tumour*

Note: *Superficial tumour is located exclusively above the superficial fascia without invasion of the fascia; deep tumour is located either exclusively beneath the superficial fascia or superficial to the fascia with invasion of or through the fascia. Retroperitoneal, mediastinal, and pelvic sarcomas are classified as deep tumours.

N – Regional Lymph Nodes

NX   Regional lymph nodes cannot be assessed
N0   No regional lymph node metastasis
N1   Regional lymph node metastasis

M – Distant Metastasis

M0   No distant metastasis
M1   Distant metastasis

pTNM Pathological Classification

The pT and pN categories correspond to the T and N categories. For pM see page 15.

G Histopathological Grading

Translation table for three- and four-grade systems to a two-grade (low grade vs high grade) system

TNM Two-grade System	Three-grade System	Four-grade System
Low grade	Grade 1	Grade 1
		Grade 2
High grade	Grade 2	Grade 3
	Grade 3	Grade 4

Note: Extraskeletal Ewing and primitive neuroectodermal tumours are classified as high grade. If grade cannot be assessed classify as low grade.

Stage Grouping

Stage IA	T1a	N0	M0	Low grade
	T1b	N0	M0	Low grade
Stage IB	T2a	N0	M0	Low grade
	T2b	N0	M0	Low grade
Stage IIA	T1a	N0	M0	High grade
	T1b	N0	M0	High grade
Stage IIB	T2a	N0	M0	High grade
Stage III	T2b	N0	M0	High grade
	Any T	N1	M0	Any G
Stage IV	Any T	Any N	M1	Any G

Note: Use low grade for GX
Use N0 for NX

Summary

Soft Tissue Sarcoma	
T1	≤5 cm
T1a	Superficial
T1b	Deep
T2	>5 cm
T2a	Superficial
T2b	Deep
N1	Regional
	Low grade
	High grade

SKIN TUMOURS

Introductory Notes

The classifications apply to carcinomas of the skin, excluding vulva (see page 197) and penis (see page 239), to malignant melanomas of the skin including eyelid and to Merkel cell carcinoma.

Anatomical Sites

The following sites are identified by ICD-O topography rubrics:

- Lip (excluding vermilion surface) (C44.0)
- Eyelid (C44.1)
- External ear (C44.2)
- Other and unspecified parts of face (C44.3)
- Scalp and neck (C44.4)
- Trunk including anal margin and perianal skin (C44.5)
- Upper limb and shoulder (C44.6)
- Lower limb and hip (C44.7)
- Scrotum (C63.2)

Each tumour type is described under the following headings:

- Rules for classification with the procedures for assessing T, N, and M categories

- Regional lymph nodes
- TNM Clinical classification
- pTNM Pathological classification
- G Histopathological grading (when applicable)
- Stage grouping
- Summary

Regional Lymph Nodes

The regional lymph nodes are those appropriate to the site of the primary tumour.

Unilateral Tumours
- *Head, neck:* Ipsilateral preauricular, submandibular, cervical, and supraclavicular lymph nodes
- *Thorax:* Ipsilateral axillary lymph nodes
- *Upper limb:* Ipsilateral epitrochlear and axillary lymph nodes
- *Abdomen, loins, and buttocks:* Ipsilateral inguinal lymph nodes
- *Lower limb:* Ipsilateral popliteal and inguinal lymph nodes
- *Anal margin and perianal skin:* Ipsilateral inguinal lymph nodes

Tumours in the Boundary Zones between the Above
The lymph nodes pertaining to the regions on both sides of the boundary zone are considered to be the regional lymph nodes.

The following 4-cm-wide bands are considered as boundary zones:

Between	Along
Right/left	Midline
Head and neck/thorax	Clavicula–acromion–upper shoulder blade edge
Thorax/upper limb	Shoulder–axilla–shoulder
Thorax/abdomen, loins, and buttocks	*Front*: middle between navel and costal arch *Back*: lower border of thoracic vertebrae (mid-transverse axis)
Abdomen, loins, and buttock/lower limb	Groin–trochanter–gluteal sulcus

Any metastasis to other than the listed regional lymph nodes is considered as M1.

Distant Metastasis

The categories M1 and pM1 may be further specified according to the following notation:

Pulmonary	PUL	Bone marrow	MAR
Osseous	OSS	Pleura	PLE
Hepatic	HEP	Peritoneum	PER
Brain	BRA	Adrenals	ADR
Lymph nodes	LYM	Skin	SKI
Others	OTH		

R Classification

See Introduction, page 19.

Carcinoma of Skin
(excluding eyelid, vulva, and penis)
(ICD-O C44.0, 2–7, C63.2)

Rules for Classification

The classification applies to carcinomas, excluding Merkel cell carcinoma. There should be histological confirmation of the disease and division of cases by histological type.

The following are the procedures for assessing T, N, and M categories:

T categories	Physical examination
N categories	Physical examination and imaging
M categories	Physical examination and imaging

Regional Lymph Nodes

The regional lymph nodes are those appropriate to the site of the primary tumour. See page 163.

TNM Clinical Classification

T – Primary Tumour

TX	Primary tumour cannot be assessed
T0	No evidence of primary tumour
Tis	Carcinoma in situ

T1   Tumour 2 cm or less in greatest dimension

T2   Tumour more than 2 cm in greatest dimension

T3   Tumour with invasion of deep structures, e.g., muscle, bone, cartilage, jaws, and orbit

T4   Tumour with direct or perineural invasion of skull base or axial skeleton

Note: In the case of multiple simultaneous tumours, the tumour with the highest T category is classified and the number of separate tumours is indicated in parentheses, e.g., T2(5)

N – Regional Lymph Nodes

NX   Regional lymph nodes cannot be assessed

N0   No regional lymph node metastasis

N1   Metastasis in a single lymph node, 3 cm or less in greatest dimension

N2   Metastasis in a single lymph node, more than 3 cm but not more than 6 cm in greatest dimension, or in multiple lymph nodes, none more than 6 cm in greatest dimension

N3   Metastasis in a lymph node, more than 6 cm in greatest dimension

M – Distant Metastasis

M0   No distant metastasis

M1   Distant metastasis

pTNM Pathological Classification

The pT and pN categories correspond to the T and N categories. For pM see page 15.

pN0 Histological examination of a regional lymphadenectomy specimen will ordinarily include 6 or more lymph nodes.

If the lymph nodes are negative, but the number ordinarily examined is not met, classify as pN0.

G Histopathological Grading

GX	Grade of differentiation cannot be assessed
G1	Well differentiated
G2	Moderately differentiated
G3	Poorly differentiated
G4	Undifferentiated

High Risk Features

Depth/Invasion	>4 mm thickness
	Clark Level IV
	Perineural invasion
	Lymphovascular invasion
Anatomic location	Primary site ear
	Primary site non-glabrous lip
Differentiation	Poorly differentiated or undifferentiated

Stage Grouping

Stage 0	Tis	N0	M0
Stage I	T1	N0	M0
Stage II	T2	N0	M0
Stage III	T3	N0	M0
	T1, T2, T3	N1	M0
Stage IV	T1, T2, T3	N2, N3	M0
	T4	Any N	M0
	Any T	Any N	M1

Note: AJCC considers Stage I tumours with more than one High Risk feature as Stage II.

Summary

Skin carcinoma

T1	≤2 cm
T2	>2 cm
T3	Deep structures
T4	Skull base, axial skeleton
N1	Single, ≤3 cm
N2	Single, >3 cm to 6 cm
	Multiple, ≤6 cm
N3	>6 cm

Carcinoma of Skin
of Eyelid
(ICD-O C44.1)

Rules of Classification

There should be histological confirmation of the disease and division of cases by histological type, e.g., basal cell, squamous cell, sebaceous carcinoma. Melanoma of the eyelid is classified with skin tumours, see page 172.

The following are procedures for assessing T, N, and M categories:

T categories	Physical examination
N categories	Physical examination
M categories	Physical examination and imaging

Regional Lymph Nodes

The regional lymph nodes are the preauricular, submandibular and cervical lymph nodes. See page 163.

TNM Clinical Classification

T – Primary Tumour

TX	Primary tumour cannot be assessed
T0	No evidence of primary tumour
Tis	Carcinoma in situ

T1   Tumour 5 mm or less in greatest dimension not invading the tarsal plate or eyelid margin

T2a   Tumour more than 5 mm, but not more than 10 mm in greatest dimension or any tumour that invades the tarsal plate or eyelid margin

T2b   Tumour more than 10 mm, but not more than 20 mm in greatest dimension, or involves full thickness eyelid

T3a   Tumour more than 20 mm in greatest dimension or any tumour that invades adjacent ocular or orbital structures or any tumour with perineural invasion

T3b   Tumour whose complete resection requires enucleation, exenteration, or bone resection

T4   Tumour is not resectable due to extensive invasion of ocular, orbital, craniofacial structures, or brain

N – Regional Lymph Nodes

NX   Regional lymph nodes cannot be assessed
N0   No regional lymph node metastasis
N1   Regional lymph node metastasis

M – Distant Metastasis

M0   No distant metastasis
M1   Distant metastasis

pTNM Pathological Classification

The pT and pN categories correspond to the T and N categories. For pM see page 15.

G Histopathological Grading

See definitions on page 167.

Stage Grouping

Stage 0	Tis	N0	M0
Stage IA	T1	N0	M0
Stage IB	T2a	N0	M0
Stage IC	T2b	N0	M0
Stage II	T3a	N0	M0
Stage IIIA	T3b	N0	M0
Stage IIIB	Any T	N1	M0
Stage IIIC	T4	Any N	M0
Stage IV	Any T	Any N	M1

Summary

Eyelid Carcinoma	
T1	≤5 mm, not in tarsal plate or lid margin
T2a	>5 to 10 mm or tarsal plate or lid margin
T2b	>10 to 20 mm or full thickness eyelid
T3a	>20 mm or adjacent ocular/orbital structures, perineural
T3b	Needs enucleation, exenteration, or bone resection
T4	Extensive invasion
N1	Regional

Malignant Melanoma of Skin
(ICD-O C44, C51.0, C60.9, C63.2)

Rules for Classification

There should be histological confirmation of the disease.

The following are the procedures for assessing N and M categories:

N categories	Physical examination and imaging
M categories	Physical examination and imaging

Regional Lymph Nodes

The regional lymph nodes are those appropriate to the site of the primary tumour. See page 163.

TNM Clinical Classification

T – Primary Tumour

The extent of the tumour is classified after excision, see pT, page 174.

N – Regional Lymph Nodes

NX   Regional lymph nodes cannot be assessed

N0   No regional lymph node metastasis

N1   Metastasis in one regional lymph node

    N1a Only microscopic metastasis (clinically occult)

    N1b Macroscopic metastasis (clinically apparent)

N2   Metastasis in two or three regional lymph nodes or satellite(s) or in-transit metastasis

    N2a Only microscopic nodal metastasis

    N2b Macroscopic nodal metastasis

    N2c Satellite(s) or in-transit metastasis *without* regional nodal metastasis

N3   Metastasis in four or more regional lymph nodes, or matted metastatic regional lymph nodes, or satellite or in-transit metastasis *with* metastasis in regional lymph node(s)

Note: Satellites are tumour nests or nodules (macro- or microscopic) within 2 cm of the primary tumour. In-transit metastasis involves skin or subcutaneous tissue more than 2 cm from the primary tumour but not beyond the regional lymph nodes.

M – Distant Metastasis

M0   No distant metastasis

M1   Distant metastasis

    M1a Skin, subcutaneous tissue or lymph node(s) beyond the regional lymph nodes

    M1b Lung

    M1c Other sites, or any site with elevated serum lactic dehydrogenase (LDH)

pTNM Pathological Classification

pT – Primary Tumour

pTX   Primary tumour cannot be assessed*
pT0   No evidence of primary tumour
pTis Melanoma in situ (Clark Level I) (atypical melanocytic hyperplasia, severe melanocytic dysplasia, not an invasive malignant lesion)

Note: *pTX includes shave biopsies and regressed melanomas.

pT1   Tumour 1 mm or less in thickness
      pT1a Clark level II or III, without ulceration
      pT1b Clark Level IV or V, or with ulceration
pT2   Tumour more than 1 mm but not more than 2 mm in thickness
      pT2a without ulceration
      pT2b with ulceration
pT3   Tumour more than 2 mm but not more than 4 mm in thickness
      pT3a without ulceration
      pT3b with ulceration
pT4   Tumour more than 4 mm in thickness
      pT4a without ulceration
      pT4b with ulceration

pN – Regional Lymph Nodes

The pN categories correspond to the N categories.

pN0   Histological examination of a regional lymphadenectomy specimen will ordinarily include 6 or more lymph nodes.

If the lymph nodes are negative, but the number ordinarily examined is not met, classify as pN0.

Classification based solely on sentinel node biopsy without subsequent lymph node dissection is designated (sn) for sentinel node, e.g., pN1(sn). See Introduction, page 13.

pM – Distant Metastasis

For pM see page 15.

Stage Grouping

Stage 0	pTis	N0	M0
Stage I	pT1	N0	M0
Stage IA	pT1a	N0	M0
Stage IB	pT1b	N0	M0
	pT2a	N0	M0
Stage IIA	pT2b	N0	M0
	pT3a	N0	M0
Stage IIB	pT3b	N0	M0
	pT4a	N0	M0
Stage IIC	pT4b	N0	M0
Stage III	Any pT	N1, N2, N3	M0
Stage IIIA	pT1a–4a	N1a, 2a	M0
Stage IIIB	pT1a–4a	N1b, 2b, 2c	M0
	pT1b–4b	N1a, 2a, 2c	M0
Stage IIIC	pT1b–4b	N1b, 2b	M0
	Any pT	N3	M0
Stage IV	Any pT	Any N	M1

Summary

Skin Malignant Melanoma	
pT1a	≤1 mm, Level II or III, no ulceration
pT1b	≤1 mm, Level IV or V, or ulceration
pT2a	>1–2 mm, no ulceration
pT2b	>1–2 mm, ulceration
pT3a	>2–4 mm, no ulceration
pT3b	>2–4 mm, ulceration
pT4a	>4 mm, no ulceration
pT4b	>4 mm, ulceration
N1	1 node
N1a	Microscopic
N1b	Macroscopic
N2	2–3 nodes or satellites/in-transit without nodes
N2a	2–3 nodes microscopic
N2b	2–3 nodes macroscopic
N2c	satellites or in-transit without nodes
N3	≥4 nodes; matted; satellites/in-transit with nodes

Merkel Cell Carcinoma of Skin
(ICD-O C44.0–9, C63.2)

Rules for Classification

The classification applies to Merkel cell carcinomas. There should be histological confirmation of the disease.

The following are the procedures for assessing T, N, and M categories:

T categories	Physical examination
N categories	Physical examination and imaging
M categories	Physical examination and imaging

Regional Lymph Nodes

The regional lymph nodes are those appropriate to the site of the primary tumour. See page 163.

TNM Clinical Classification

T – Primary Tumour

TX	Primary tumour cannot be assessed
T0	No evidence of primary tumour
Tis	Carcinoma in situ

T1	Tumour 2 cm or less in greatest dimension
T2	Tumour more than 2 cm but not more than 5 cm in greatest dimension
T3	Tumour more than 5 cm in greatest dimension
T4	Tumour invades deep extradermal structures, i.e., cartilage, skeletal muscle, fascia, or bone

N – Regional Lymph Nodes

NX	Regional lymph nodes cannot be assessed
N0	No regional lymph node metastasis
N1	Regional lymph node metastasis
	N1a Microscopic metastasis (clinically occult: cN0 + pN1)
	N1b Macroscopic metastasis (clinically apparent: cN1 + pN1)
N2	In-transit metastasis*

Note: *In-transit metastasis: a tumour distinct from the primary lesion and located between the primary lesion and the draining regional lymph nodes or distal to the primary lesion.

M – Distant Metastasis

M0	No distant metastasis
M1	Distant metastasis
	M1a Skin, subcutaneous tissues or non-regional lymph node(s)
	M1b Lung
	M1c Other site(s)

pTNM Pathological Classification

The pT and pN categories correspond to the T and N categories. For pM see page 163.

pN0   Histological examination of a regional lymphadenectomy specimen will ordinarily include 6 or more lymph nodes.

If the lymph nodes are negative, but the number ordinarily examined is not met, classify as pN0.

Histopathological Grading

Not applicable.

Stage Grouping

Stage 0	Tis	N0	M0
Stage I	T1	N0	M0
Stage IA	T1	pN0	M0
Stage IB	T1	cN0	M0
Stage IIA	T2, T3	pN0	M0
Stage IIB	T2, T3	cN0	M0
Stage IIC	T4	N0	M0
Stage IIIA	Any T	N1a	M0
Stage IIIB	Any T	N1b, N2	M0
Stage IV	Any T	Any N	M1

Summary

Merkel Cell Carcinoma

T1	≤2 cm
T2	>2 cm to 5 cm
T3	>5 cm
T4	Deep extradermal structures (cartilage, skeletal muscle, fascia, bone)
N1	Regional
N1a	Microscopic
N1b	Macroscopic
N2	In-transit metastasis
M1	Distant metastasis
M1a	Skin, subcutaneous tissues or non-regional lymph nodes
M1b	Lung
M1c	Other site(s)

BREAST TUMOURS
(ICD-O C50)

Introductory Notes

The site is described under the following headings:

- Rules for classification with the procedures for assessing T, N, and M categories; additional methods may be used when they enhance the accuracy of appraisal before treatment
- Anatomical subsites
- Definition of the regional lymph nodes
- TNM Clinical classification
- pTNM Pathological classification
- G Histopathological grading
- R Classification
- Stage grouping
- Summary

Rules for Classification

The classification applies to carcinomas and concerns the male as well as the female breast. There should be histological confirmation of the disease. The anatomical subsite of origin should be recorded but is not considered in classification.

In the case of multiple simultaneous primary tumours in one breast, the tumour with the highest T category should be used for classification. Simultaneous *bilateral* breast cancers should be classified independently to permit division of cases by histological type.

The following are the procedures for assessing T, N, and M categories:

T categories	Physical examination and imaging, e.g., mammography
N categories	Physical examination and imaging
M categories	Physical examination and imaging

Anatomical Subsites

1. Nipple (C50.0)
2. Central portion (C50.1)
3. Upper-inner quadrant (C50.2)
4. Lower-inner quadrant (C50.3)
5. Upper-outer quadrant (C50.4)
6. Lower-outer quadrant (C50.5)
7. Axillary tail (C50.6)

Regional Lymph Nodes

The regional lymph nodes are:

1. *Axillary* (ipsilateral): interpectoral (Rotter) nodes and lymph nodes along the axillary vein and its tributaries, which may be divided into the following levels:
   - *(i)* *Level I* (low-axilla): lymph nodes lateral to the lateral border of pectoralis minor muscle
   - *(ii)* *Level II* (mid-axilla): lymph nodes between the medial and lateral borders of the pectoralis minor muscle and the interpectoral (Rotter) lymph nodes
   - (iii) Level III (apical axilla): apical lymph nodes and those medial to the medial margin of the pectoralis minor muscle, excluding those designated as subclavicular or infraclavicular

Note: Intramammary lymph nodes are coded as axillary lymph nodes Level I.

2. *Infraclavicular (subclavicular)* (ipsilateral)
3. *Internal mammary* (ipsilateral): lymph nodes in the intercostal spaces along the edge of the sternum in the endothoracic fascia
4. *Supraclavicular* (ipsilateral)

Note: Any other lymph node metastasis is coded as a distant metastasis (M1), including cervical or contralateral internal mammary lymph nodes.

TNM Clinical Classification

T – Primary Tumour

TX	Primary tumour cannot be assessed
T0	No evidence of primary tumour
Tis	Carcinoma in situ

Tis (DCIS)   Ductal carcinoma in situ
Tis (LCIS)   Lobular carcinoma in situ
Tis (Paget) Paget disease of the nipple not associated with invasive carcinoma and/or carcinoma in situ (DCIS and/or LCIS) in the underlying breast parenchyma. Carcinomas in the breast parenchyma associated with Paget disease are categorized based on the size and characteristics of the parenchymal disease, although the presence of Paget disease should still be noted.

T1   Tumour 2 cm or less in greatest dimension
          T1mi Microinvasion 0.1 cm or less in greatest dimension*

Note: *Microinvasion is the extension of cancer cells beyond the basement membrane into the adjacent tissues with no focus more than 0.1 cm in greatest dimension. When there are multiple foci of microinvasion, the size of only the largest focus is used to classify the microinvasion. (Do not use the sum of all individual foci.) The presence of multiple foci of microinvasion should be noted, as it is with multiple larger invasive carcinomas.

          T1a More than 0.1 cm but not more than 0.5 cm in greatest dimension
          T1b More than 0.5 cm but not more than 1 cm in greatest dimension
          T1c More than 1 cm but not more than 2 cm in greatest dimension
T2   Tumour more than 2 cm but not more than 5 cm in greatest dimension
T3   Tumour more than 5 cm in greatest dimension
T4   Tumour of any size with direct extension to chest wall and/or to skin (ulceration or skin nodules)

Note: Invasion of the dermis alone does not qualify as T4. Chest wall includes ribs, intercostal muscles, and serratus anterior muscle but not pectoral muscle.

T4a Extension to chest wall (does not include pectoralis muscle invasion only)

T4b Ulceration, ipsilateral satellite skin nodules, or skin oedema (including peau d'orange)

T4c Both 4a and 4b, above

T4d Inflammatory carcinoma

Note: Inflammatory carcinoma of the breast is characterized by diffuse, brawny induration of the skin with an erysipeloid edge, usually with no underlying mass. If the skin biopsy is negative and there is no localized measurable primary cancer, the T category is pTX when pathologically staging a clinical inflammatory carcinoma (T4d). Dimpling of the skin, nipple retraction, or other skin changes, except those in T4b and T4d, may occur in T1, T2, or T3 without affecting the classification.

N – Regional Lymph Nodes

NX Regional lymph nodes cannot be assessed (e.g., previously removed)

N0 No regional lymph node metastasis

N1 Metastasis in movable ipsilateral Level I, II axillary lymph node(s)

N2 Metastasis in ipsilateral Level I, II axillary lymph node(s) that are clinically fixed or matted; or in clinically detected* ipsilateral internal mammary lymph node(s) in the *absence* of clinically evident axillary lymph node metastasis

N2a Metastasis in axillary lymph node(s) fixed to one another (matted) or to other structures

N2b Metastasis only in clinically detected* internal mammary lymph node(s) and in the *absence* of clinically detected axillary lymph node metastasis

N3 Metastasis in ipsilateral infraclavicular (Level III axillary) lymph node(s) with or without Level I, II axillary lymph node involvement; or in clinically detected* ipsilateral internal mammary lymph node(s) with clinically evident Level I, II axillary lymph node metastasis; or metastasis in ipsilateral supraclavicular lymph node(s) with or without axillary or internal mammary lymph node involvement

N3a Metastasis in infraclavicular lymph node(s)

N3b Metastasis in internal mammary and axillary lymph nodes

N3c Metastasis in supraclavicular lymph node(s)

Note: *Clinically detected is defined as detected by clinical examination or by imaging studies (excluding lymphoscintigraphy) and having characteristics highly suspicious for malignancy or a presumed pathological macrometastasis based on fine-needle aspiration biopsy with cytological examination. Confirmation of clinically detected metastatic disease by fine-needle aspiration without excision biopsy is designated with an (f) suffix, e.g., cN3a(f).

Excisional biopsy of a lymph node or biopsy of a sentinel node, in the absence of assignment of a pT, is classified as a clinical N, e.g., cN1. Pathological classification (pN) is used for excision or sentinel lymph node biopsy only in conjunction with a pathological T assignment.

M – Distant Metastasis

M0 No distant metastasis

M1 Distant metastasis

The categories M1 and pM1 may be further specified according to the following notation:

Pulmonary	PUL	Bone marrow	MAR
Osseous	OSS	Pleura	PLE
Hepatic	HEP	Peritoneum	PER
Brain	BRA	Adrenals	ADR
Lymph nodes	LYM	Skin	SKI
Others	OTH		

pTNM Pathological Classification

pT – Primary Tumour

The pathological classification requires the examination of the primary carcinoma with no gross tumour at the margins of resection. A case can be classified pT if there is only microscopic tumour in a margin.

The pT categories correspond to the T categories.

Note: When classifying pT the tumour size is a measurement of the invasive component. If there is a large in situ component (e.g., 4 cm) and a small invasive component (e.g., 0.5 cm), the tumour is coded pT1a.

pN – Regional Lymph Nodes

The pathological classification requires the resection and examination of at least the low axillary lymph nodes (Level I) (see page 183.). Such a resection will ordinarily include 6 or more lymph nodes.

If the lymph nodes are negative, but the number ordinarily examined is not met, classify as pN0.

pNX   Regional lymph nodes cannot be assessed (e.g., previously removed, or not removed for pathological study)

pN0   No regional lymph node metastasis*

Note: *Isolated tumour cell clusters (ITC) are single tumour cells or small clusters of cells not more than 0.2 mm in greatest extent that can be detected by routine H&E stains or immunohistochemistry. An additional criterion has been proposed to include a cluster of fewer than 200 cells in a single histological cross-section. Nodes containing only ITCs are excluded from the total positive node count for purposes of N classification and should be included in the total number of nodes evaluated. See Introduction, page 13.

pN1   Micrometastasis; or metastasis in 1–3 axillary ipsilateral lymph nodes; and/or in internal mammary nodes with metastasis detected by sentinel lymph node biopsy but not clinically detected[1]

   pN1mi   Micrometastasis (larger than 0.2 mm and/or more than 200 cells, but none larger than 2.0 mm)

   pN1a   Metastasis in 1–3 axillary lymph node(s), including at least 1 larger than 2 mm in greatest dimension

   pN1b   Internal mammary lymph nodes with microscopic or macroscopic metastasis detected by sentinel lymph node biopsy but not clinically detected[1]

   pN1c   Metastasis in 1–3 axillary lymph nodes and internal mammary lymph nodes with microscopic or macroscopic metastasis detected by sentinel lymph node biopsy but not clinically detected[1]

pN2   Metastasis in 4–9 ipsilateral axillary lymph nodes, or in clinically detected[1] ipsilateral internal mammary lymph node(s) in the absence of axillary lymph node metastasis

pN2a   Metastasis in 4–9 axillary lymph nodes, including at least one that is larger than 2 mm

pN2b   Metastasis in clinically detected[1] internal mammary lymph node(s), in the *absence* of axillary lymph node metastasis

pN3   Metastasis as described below:

pN3a   Metastasis in 10 or more axillary lymph nodes (at least one larger than 2 mm) *or* metastasis in infraclavicular lymph nodes

pN3b   Metastasis in clinically detected[1] internal ipsilateral mammary lymph node(s) in the *presence* of positive axillary lymph node(s); or metastasis in more than 3 axillary lymph nodes *and* in internal mammary lymph nodes with microscopic or macroscopic metastasis detected by sentinel lymph node biopsy but not clinically detected

pN3c   Metastasis in ipsilateral supraclavicular lymph node(s)

Post-treatment ypN:

- Post-treatment ypN should be evaluated as for clinical (pretreatment) N methods above. The modifier sn is used only if a sentinel node evaluation was performed after treatment. If no subscript is attached, it is assumed the axillary nodal evaluation was by axillary node dissection.

- The X classification will be used (ypNX) if no yp post-treatment SN or axillary dissection was performed
- N categories are the same as those used for pN.

Note: 1. *Clinically detected* is defined as detected by imaging studies (excluding lymphoscintigraphy) or by clinical examination and having characteristics highly suspicious for malignancy or a presumed pathological macrometastasis based on fine-needle aspiration biopsy with cytological examination.

Not clinically detected is defined as not detected by imaging studies (excluding lymphoscintigraphy) or not detected by clinical examination.

pM – Distant Metastasis

For pM see page 15.

G Histopathological Grading

For histopathological grading of invasive carcinoma see: Elston CW, Ellis IO. Pathological prognostic factors in breast cancer. I. The value of histological grade in breast cancer: experience from a large study with long-term follow-up. *Histopathology* 1991; 19:403–410.

R Classification

See Introduction, page 19.

Stage Grouping

Stage 0	Tis	N0	M0
Stage IA	T1*	N0	M0
Stage IB	T0, T1*	N1mi	M0
Stage IIA	T0, T1*	N1	M0
	T2	N0	M0
Stage IIB	T2	N1	M0
	T3	N0	M0
Stage IIIA	T0, T1*, T2	N2	M0
	T3	N1, N2	M0
Stage IIIB	T4	N0, N1, N2	M0
Stage IIIC	Any T	N3	M0
Stage IV	Any T	Any N	M1

Note: *T1 includes T1mi.

Summary

Breast			
Tis	in situ		
T1	≤2 cm		
T1mi	≤0.1 cm		
T1a	>0.1 cm to 0.5 cm		
T1b	>0.5 cm to 1.0 cm		
T1c	>1.0 cm to 2.0 cm		
T2	>2 cm to 5 cm		
T3	>5 cm		
T4	Chest wall/skin ulceration, skin nodules, inflammatory		
T4a	Chest wall		
T4b	Skin ulceration, satellite skin nodules, skin oedema		
T4c	Both T4a and T4b		
T4d	Inflammatory carcinoma		
N1	Movable axillary	pN1mi	Micrometastasis >0.2 mm to 2 mm
		pN1a	1–3 axillary nodes
		pN1b	Internal mammary nodes with microscopic/macroscopic metastasis by sentinel node biopsy but not clinically detected
		pN1c	1–3 axillary nodes and internal mammary nodes and internal mammary nodes with microscopic/macroscopic metastasis by sentinel node biopsy but not clinically detected

N2a	Fixed axillary	pN2a	4–9 axillary nodes
N2b	Internal mammary clinically apparent	pN2b	Internal mammary nodes, clinically detected, without axillary nodes
N3a	Infra-clavicular	pN3a	⩾10 axillary nodes or infraclavicular
N3b	Internal mammary and axillary	pN3b	Internal mammary nodes, clinically detected, with node(s) or >3 axillary nodes and internal axillary mammary nodes with microscopic metastasis by sentinel node biopsy but not clinically detected
N3c	Supra-clavicular	pN3c	Supraclavicular

GYNAECOLOGICAL TUMOURS

The following sites are included:

- Vulva
- Vagina
- Cervix uteri
- Corpus uteri
  - Endometrium
  - Uterine sarcomas
- Ovary
- Fallopian tube
- Gestational trophoblastic tumours

Cervix uteri and corpus uteri were among the first sites to be classified by the TNM system. Originally, carcinoma of the cervix uteri was staged following the rules suggested by the Radiological Sub-Commission of the Cancer Commission of the Health Organization of the 'League of Nations'. These rules were then adopted, with minor modifications, by the newly formed Fédération Internationale de Gynécologie et d'Obstétrique (FIGO). Finally, UICC brought them into the TNM in order to correspond to the FIGO stages. FIGO, UICC, and AJCC work in close collaboration in the revision process.

Reference:

Pecotelli S. Revised FIGO staging for carcinoma of the Gulva cervix and endometrium. Int J Gynecol Obstet 2009, 105: 103–104

Each site is described under the following headings:

- Rules for classification with the procedures for assessing T, N, and M categories; additional methods may be used when they enhance the accuracy of appraisal before treatment
- Anatomical subsites where appropriate
- Definition of the regional lymph nodes
- TNM Clinical classification
- pTNM Pathological classification
- G Histopathological grading where applicable
- Stage grouping
- Summary

Distant Metastasis

The categories M1 and pM1 may be further specified according to the following notation:

Pulmonary	PUL	Bone marrow	MAR
Osseous	OSS	Pleura	PLE
Hepatic	HEP	Peritoneum	PER
Brain	BRA	Adrenals	ADR
Lymph nodes	LYM	Skin	SKI
Others	OTH		

Histopathological Grading

The definitions of the G categories apply to all carcinomas. These are:

G Histopathological Grading

GX   Grade of differentiation cannot be assessed
G1   Well differentiated

G2	Moderately differentiated
G3	Poorly differentiated or undifferentiated

R Classification

See Introduction, page 19.

Vulva
(ICD-O C51)

The definitions of the T, N, and M categories correspond to the FIGO stages. Both systems are included for comparison.

Rules for Classification

The classification applies to primary carcinomas of the vulva. There should be histological confirmation of the disease.

A carcinoma of the vulva that has extended to the vagina is classified as carcinoma of the vulva.

The following are the procedures for assessing T, N, and M categories:

T categories	Physical examination, endoscopy, and imaging
N categories	Physical examination and imaging
M categories	Physical examination and imaging

The FIGO stages are based on surgical staging. (TNM stages are based on clinical and/or pathological classification.)

Regional Lymph Nodes

The regional lymph nodes are the inguinofemoral (groin) nodes.

TNM Clinical Classification

T – Primary Tumour

TX   Primary tumour cannot be assessed
T0   No evidence of primary tumour
Tis   Carcinoma in situ (preinvasive carcinoma), intraepithelial neoplasia Grade III (VIN III)

T1   Tumour confined to vulva or vulva and perineum

      T1a Tumour 2 cm or less in greatest dimension and with stromal invasion no greater than 1.0 mm[1]

      T1b Tumour greater than 2 cm or with stromal invasion greater than 1 mm[1]

T2   Tumour of any size with extension to adjacent perineal structures: lower third urethra, lower third vagina, anus

T3[2] Tumour of any size with extension to the following structures: upper 2/3 urethra, upper 2/3 vagina, bladder mucosa, rectal mucosa; or fixed to pelvic bone

Notes: 1. The depth of invasion is defined as the measurement of the tumour from the epithelial–stromal junction of the adjacent most superficial dermal papilla to the deepest point of invasion.
        2. T3 is not used by FIGO. They label it T4.

N – Regional Lymph Nodes

NX   Regional lymph nodes cannot be assessed
N0   No regional lymph node metastasis
N1   Regional lymph node metastasis with the following features:

N1a 1–2 lymph node metastasis each less than 5 mm

N1b 1 lymph node metastases 5 mm or greater

N2 Regional lymph node metastasis with the following features:

N2a 3 or more lymph node metastases each less than 5 mm

N2b 2 or more lymph node metastases 5 mm or greater

N2c Lymph node metastasis with extracapsular spread

N3 Fixed or ulcerated regional lymph node metastasis

M – Distant Metastasis

M0 No distant metastasis

M1 Distant metastasis (including pelvic lymph node metastasis)

pTNM Pathological Classification

The pT and pN categories correspond to the T and N categories. For pM see page 15.

pN0 Histological examination of an inguinofemoral lymphadenectomy specimen will ordinarily include 6 or more lymph nodes.

If the lymph nodes are negative, but the number ordinarily examined is not met, classify as pN0. (FIGO considers such cases as pNX)

G Histopathological Grading

See definitions on page 195.

Stage Grouping

Stage 0*	Tis	N0	M0
Stage I	T1	N0	M0
Stage IA	T1a	N0	M0
Stage IB	T1b	N0	M0
Stage II	T2	N0	M0
Stage IIIA	T1, T2	N1a, N1b	M0
Stage IIIB	T1, T2	N2a, N2b	M0
Stage IIIC	T1, T2	N2c	M0
Stage IVA	T1, T2	N3	M0
	T3	Any N	M0
Stage IVB	Any T	Any N	M1

Note: * FIGO no longer includes stage 0 (Tis).

Summary

TNM	Vulva	FIGO
T1	Confined to vulva/perineum	I
T1a	≤2 cm with stromal invasion ≤1.0 mm	IA
T1b	>2 cm or stromal invasion >1.0 mm	IB
T2	Lower urethra/vagina/anus	II
T3	Upper urethra/vagina, bladder rectal/mucosa, fixed to pelvic bone	IVA
N1a	1–2 nodes <5 mm	IIIA
N1b	1 node ≥5 mm	IIIA
N2a	3 or more nodes <5 mm	IIIB
N2b	2 or more nodes ≥5 mm	IIIB
N2c	Extracapsular spread	IIIC
N3	Fixed	IVA
M1	Distant	IVB

Vagina
(ICD-O C52)

The definitions of the T and M categories correspond to the FIGO stages. Both systems are included for comparison.

Rules for Classification

The classification applies to primary carcinomas only. Tumours present in the vagina as secondary growths from either genital or extragenital sites are excluded. A tumour that has extended to the portio and reached the external os (orifice of uterus) is classified as carcinoma of the cervix. A vaginal carcinoma occurring 5 years after successful treatment (complete response) of a carcinoma of the cervix uteri is considered a primary vaginal carcinoma. A tumour involving the vulva is classified as carcinoma of the vulva. There should be histological confirmation of the disease.

The following are the procedures for assessing T, N, and M categories:

T categories	Physical examination, endoscopy, and imaging
N categories	Physical examination and imaging
M categories	Physical examination and imaging

The FIGO stages are based on surgical staging. (TNM stages are based on clinical and/or pathological classification.)

Regional Lymph Nodes

Upper two-thirds of vagina: the pelvic nodes including obturator, internal iliac (hypogastric), external iliac, and pelvic nodes, NOS.

Lower third of vagina: the inguinal and femoral nodes.

TNM Clinical Classification

T – Primary Tumour

TNM Categories	FIGO Stages	
TX		Primary tumour cannot be assessed
T0		No evidence of primary tumour
Tis	[1]	Carcinoma in situ (preinvasive carcinoma)
T1	I	Tumour confined to vagina
T2	II	Tumour invades paravaginal tissues (paracolpium)
T3	III	Tumour extends to pelvic wall
T4	IVA	Tumour invades *mucosa* of bladder or rectum, or extends beyond the true pelvis[2]

Notes: 1. FIGO no longer includes stage 0 (Tis).
2. The presence of bullous oedema is not sufficient evidence to classify a tumour as T4

M1	IVB	Distant metastasis

N — Regional Lymph Nodes

NX   Regional lymph nodes cannot be assessed
N0   No regional lymph node metastasis
N1   Regional lymph node metastasis

M — Distant Metastasis

M0   No distant metastasis
M1   Distant metastasis

TNM Pathological Classification

The pT and pN categories correspond to the T and N categories. For pM see page 15.

pN0   Histological examination of an inguinal lymphadenectomy specimen will ordinarily include 6 or more lymph nodes; a pelvic lymphadenectomy specimen will ordinarily include 6 or more lymph nodes.

   If the lymph nodes are negative, but the number ordinarily examined is not met, classify as pN0. (FIGO considers such cases pNX).

G Histopathological Grading

See definitions on page 195.

Stage Grouping

Stage 0	Tis	N0	M0
Stage I	T1	N0	M0
Stage II	T2	N0	M0
Stage III	T3	N0	M0
	T1, T2, T3	N1	M0
Stage IVA	T4	Any N	M0
Stage IVB	Any T	Any N	M1

Summary

TNM	Vagina	FIGO
T1	Vaginal wall	I
T2	Paravaginal tissue	II
T3	Pelvic wall	III
T4	Mucosa of bladder/rectum, beyond pelvis	IVA
N1	Regional	
M1	Distant metastasis	IVB

Cervix Uteri
(ICD-O C53)

The definitions of the T and M categories correspond to the FIGO stages. Both systems are included for comparison.

Rules for Classification

The classification applies only to carcinomas. There should be histological confirmation of the disease.

The following are the procedures for assessing T, N, and M categories:

T categories	Clinical examination and imaging*
N categories	Clinical examination and imaging
M categories	Clinical examination and imaging

Note: *The use of diagnostic imaging techniques to assess the size of the primary tumour is encouraged but is not mandatory. Other investigations, e.g., examination under anaesthesia, cystoscopy, sigmoidoscopy, intravenous pyelography, are optional and no longer mandatory.

The FIGO stages are based on clinical staging. Some Stage I subdivisions require histological examination of the cervix. (TNM stages are based on clinical and/or pathological classification.)

Anatomical Subsites

1. Endocervix (C53.0)
2. Exocervix (C53.1)

Regional Lymph Nodes

The regional lymph nodes are the paracervical, parametrial, hypogastric (internal iliac, obturator), common and external iliac, presacral, and lateral sacral nodes. Para-aortic nodes are not regional.

TNM Clinical Classification

T – Primary Tumour

TNM Categories	FIGO Stages	
TX		Primary tumour cannot be assessed
T0		No evidence of primary tumour
Tis	[1]	Carcinoma in situ (preinvasive carcinoma)
T1	I	Tumour confined to the cervix (extension to corpus should be disregarded)
T1a[2]	IA	Invasive carcinoma diagnosed only by microscopy. Stromal invasion with a maximal depth of 5.0 mm measured from the base of the epithelium and a horizontal spread of 7.0 mm or less[3]

T1a1	IA1	Measured stromal invasion 3.0 mm or less in depth and 7.0 mm or less in horizontal spread
T1a2	IA2	Measured stromal invasion more than 3.0 mm and not more than 5.0 mm with a horizontal spread of 7.0 mm or less

Note: The depth of invasion should be taken from the base of the epithelium, either surface or glandular, from which it originates. The depth of invasion is defined as the measurement of the tumour from the epithelial–stromal junction of the adjacent most superficial papillae to the deepest point of invasion.

Vascular space involvement, venous or lymphatic, does not affect classification.

T1b	IB	Clinically visible lesion confined to the cervix or microscopic lesion greater than T1a/IA2
T1b1	IB1	Clinically visible lesion 4.0 cm or less in greatest dimension
T1b2	IB2	Clinically visible lesion more than 4.0 cm in greatest dimension
T2	II	Tumour invades beyond uterus but not to pelvic wall or to lower third of vagina
T2a	IIA	Tumour without parametrial invasion
T2a1	IIA1	Clinically visible lesion 4.0 cm or less in greatest dimension
T2a2	IIA2	Clinically visible lesion more than 4.0 cm in greatest dimension
T2b	IIB	Tumour with parametrial invasion

T3	III	Tumour extends to pelvic wall, involves lower third of vagina, causes hydronephrosis or non-functioning kidney
T3a	IIIA	Tumour involves lower third of vagina
T3b	IIIB	Tumour extends to pelvic wall, causes hydronephrosis or non-functioning kidney
T4	IVA	Tumour invades mucosa of the bladder or rectum, or extends beyond true pelvis[4,5]

Notes:

[1] FIGO no longer includes Stage 0 (Tis).

[2] All macroscopically visible lesions even with superficial invasion are T1b/IB.

[3] Vascular space involvement, venous or lymphatic, does not affect classification.

[4] Bullous oedema is not sufficient to classify a tumour as T4.

[5] Invasion of bladder or rectal mucosa should be biopsy proven according to FIGO

N – Regional lymph nodes

NX   Regional lymph nodes cannot be assessed
N0   No regional lymph node metastasis
N1   Regional lymph node metastasis

M – Distant Metastasis

M0   No distant metastasis
M1   Distant metastasis (includes inguinal lymph nodes and intraperitoneal disease except metastasis to pelvic serosa). It excludes metastasis to vagina, pelvic serosa, and adnexa

pTNM Pathological Classification

The pT and pN categories correspond to the T and N categories. For pM see page 15.

pN0   Histological examination of a pelvic lymphadenectomy specimen will ordinarily include 6 or more lymph nodes.

If the lymph nodes are negative, but the number ordinarily examined is not met, classify as pN0.

G Histopathological Grading

See definitions on page 195

Stage Grouping

Stage 0*	Tis	N0	M0
Stage I	T1	N0	M0
Stage IA	T1a	N0	M0
Stage IA1	T1a1	N0	M0
Stage IA2	T1a2	N0	M0
Stage IB	T1b	N0	M0
Stage IB1	T1b1	N0	M0
Stage IB2	T1b2	N0	M0
Stage II	T2	N0	M0
Stage IIA	T2a	N0	M0
Stage IIA1	T2a1	N0	M0
Stage IIA2	T2a2	N0	M0
Stage IIB	T2b	N0	M0
Stage III	T3	N0	M0
Stage IIIA	T3a	N0	M0
Stage IIIB	T3b	Any N	M0
	T1, T2, T3	N1	M0
Stage IVA	T4	Any N	M0
Stage IVB	Any T	Any N	M1

Note: *FIGO no longer includes stage 0 (Tis)

Summary

TNM	Cervix Uteri	FIGO
Tis	In situ	–
T1	Confined to uterus	I
T1a	Diagnosed only by microscopy	IA
T1a1	Depth ≤3 mm, horizontal spread ≤7 mm	IA1
T1a2	Depth >3–5 mm, horizontal spread ≤7 mm	IA2
T1b	Clinically visible or microscopic lesion greater than T1a2	IB
T1b1	≤4 cm	IB1
T1b2	>4 cm	IB2
T2	Beyond uterus but not pelvic wall or lower third vagina	II
T2a	No parametrium	IIA
T2a1	≤4 cm	IIA1
T2a2	>4 cm	IIA2
T2b	Parametrium	IIB
T3	Lower third vagina/pelvic wall/hydronephrosis	III
T3a	Lower third vagina	IIIA
T3b	Pelvic wall/hydronephrosis	IIIB
T4	Mucosa of bladder/rectum; beyond true pelvis	IVA
N1	Regional	
M1	Distant metastasis	IVB

Uterus - Endometrium
(ICD-O C54.1,55)

The definitions of the T, N, and M categories correspond to the FIGO stages. Both systems are included for comparison.

Rules for Classification

The classification applies to endometrial carcinomas and carcinosarcomas (malignant mixed mesodermal tumours). There should be histological verification with subdivision by histological type and grading of the carcinomas. The diagnosis should be based on examination of specimens taken by endometrial biopsy.

The following are the procedures for assessing T, N, and M categories:

T categories	Physical examination and imaging including urography and cystoscopy
N categories	Physical examination and imaging including urography
M categories	Physical examination and imaging

The FIGO stages are based on surgical staging. (TNM stages are based on clinical and/or pathological classification.)

Anatomical Subsites

1. Isthmus uteri (C54.0)
2. Fundus uteri (C54.3)
3. Endometrium (C54.1)

Regional Lymph Nodes

The regional lymph nodes are the pelvic (hypogastric [obturator, internal iliac], common and external iliac, parametrial, and sacral) and the para-aortic nodes.

TNM Clinical Classification

T – Primary Tumour

TNM Categories	FIGO Stages	
TX		Primary tumour cannot be assessed
T0		No evidence of primary tumour
Tis		Carcinoma in situ (preinvasive carcinoma)
T1	I[1]	Tumour confined to the corpus uteri[1]
T1a	IA[1]	Tumour limited to endometrium or invading less than half of myo-metrium
T1b	IB	Tumour invades one half or more of myometrium
T2	II	Tumour invades cervical stroma, but does not extend beyond the uterus

T3 and/or N1	III	Local and/or regional spread as specified below:
T3a	IIIA	Tumour invades the serosa of the corpus uteri or adnexae (direct extension or metastasis)
T3b	IIIB	Vaginal or parametrial involvement (direct extension or metastasis)
N1	IIIC	Metastasis to pelvic or para-aortic lymph nodes[2]
	IIIC1	Metastasis to pelvic lymph nodes
	IIIC2	Metastasis to para-aortic lymph nodes with or without metastasis to pelvic lymph nodes
T4	IVA	Tumour invades bladder/bowel mucosa[3]
M1	IVB	**Note:** The presence of bullous oedema is not sufficient evidence to classify as T4. This lesion should be confirmed by biopsy.

Notes:

1. Endocervical glandular involvement only should now be considered as Stage I.
2. Positive cytology has to be reported separately without changing the stage.
3. The presence of bullous oedema is not sufficient evidence to classify as T4.

N – Regional Lymph Nodes

NX   Regional lymph nodes cannot be assessed
N0   No regional lymph node metastasis
N1   Regional lymph node metastasis

M – Distant Metastasis

M0 No distant metastasis
M1 Distant metastasis (excluding metastasis to vagina, pelvic serosa, or adnexa, including metastasis to inguinal lymph nodes, intra-abdominal lymph nodes other than para-aortic or pelvic nodes)

pTNM Pathological Classification

The pT and pN categories correspond to the T and N categories. For pM see page 15.

pN0 Histological examination of a pelvic lymphadenectomy specimen will ordinarily include 6 or more lymph nodes.

If the lymph nodes are negative, but the number ordinarily examined is not met, classify as pN0. (FIGO considers such cases as pNX).

G Histopathological Grading

For histopathological grading use G1, G2, or G3. For details see:

Creasman WT, Odicino F, Maisoneuve P, et al. FIGO Annual Report on the results of treatment in gynaecological cancer. Vol. 26. Carcinoma of the corpus uteri. *Int J Gynecol Obstet* 2006; 95, Suppl 1:105–143.

Stage Grouping

Stage IA	T1a	N0	M0
Stage IB	T1b	N0	M0
Stage II	T2	N0	M0
Stage IIIA	T3a	N0	M0
Stage IIIB	T3b	N0	M0
Stage IIIC	T1, T2, T3	N1	M0
Stage IVA	T4	Any N	M0
Stage IVB	Any T	Any N	M1

Summary

TNM	Corpus Uteri	FIGO
T1	Confined to corpus (includes endocervical glands)	I
T1a	Tumour limited to endometrium or less than one-half of myometrium	IA
T1b	One-half or more of myometrium	IB
T2	Invades cervix	II
T3 and/or N1	Local or regional as specified below	III
T3a	Serosa/adnexa	IIIA
T3b	Vaginal/parametrial	IIIB
N1	Regional lymph node metastasis	IIIC
T4	Mucosa of bladder/bowel	IVA
M1	Distant metastasis	IVB

Uterus - Uterine Sarcomas
(leiomyosarcoma, endometrial stromal sarcoma, adenosarcoma)
(ICD-0 53, 54 (except 54.1))

The definitions of the T, N, and M categories correspond to the FIGO stages. Both systems are included for comparison.

References:

Prat J. FIGO staging for uterine sarcomas. *Int J Gynaecol Obstet* 2009; 104:177–178.

FIGO Committee on Gyn Onc Report. FIGO staging for uterine sarcomas. *Int J Gynaecol Obstet* 2009; 104:179.

Rules for Classification

The classification applies to sarcomas except for carcinosarcoma, which is classified along with carcinoma of the endometrium. There should be histological confirmation and division of cases by histological type.

The following are the procedures for assessing T, N, and M categories:

T categories	Physical examination and imaging
N categories	Physical examination and imaging
M categories	Physical examination and imaging

The FIGO stages are based on surgical staging. (TNM stages are based on clinical and/or pathological classification.)

Anatomical Subsites

1. Cervix uteri (C53)
2. Isthmus uteri (C54.0)
3. Fundus uteri (C54.3)

Histological Types of Tumours

Leiomyosarcoma	8890/3
Endometrial stromal sarcoma	8930/3
Adenosarcoma	8933/3

Regional Lymph Nodes

The regional lymph nodes are the pelvic (hypogastric [obturator, internal iliac], common and external iliac, parametrial, and sacral) and the para-aortic nodes.

TNM Clinical Classification

Leiomyosarcoma, Endometrial stromal sarcoma

T – Primary Tumour

TNM categories	FIGO Stage	Definition
T1	I	Tumour limited to the uterus
T1a	IA	Tumour 5 cm or less in greatest dimension
T1b	IB	Tumour more than 5 cm in greatest dimension
T2	II	Tumour extends beyond the uterus, within the pelvis

T2a	IIA	Tumour involves adnexa
T2b	IIB	Tumour involves other pelvic tissues
T3	III	Tumour involves abdominal tissues
T3a	IIIA	One site
T3b	IIIB	More than one site
N1	IIIC	Metastasis to regional lymph nodes
T4	IVA	Tumour invades bladder or rectal mucosa
M1	IVB	Distant metastasis

Note: Simultaneous tumours of the uterine corpus and ovary/pelvis in association with ovarian/pelvic endometriosis should be classified as independent primary tumours.

TNM Clinical Classification

Adenosarcoma

T – Primary Tumour

TNM categories	FIGO Stage	Definition
T1	I	Tumour limited to the uterus
T1a	IA	Tumour limited to the endometrium/ endocervix
T1b	IB	Tumour invades less than half of the myometrium
T1c	IC	Tumour invades one half or more of the myometrium
T2	II	Tumour extends beyond the uterus, within the pelvis

T2a	IIA	Tumour involves adnexa
T2b	IIB	Tumour involves other pelvic tissues
T3	III	Tumour involves abdominal tissues
T3a	IIIA	One site
T3b	IIIB	More than one site
N1	IIIC	Metastasis to regional lymph nodes
T4	IVA	Tumour invades bladder or rectal mucosa
M1	IVB	Distant metastasis

Note: Simultaneous tumours of the uterine corpus and ovary/ pelvis in association with ovarian/pelvic endometriosis should be classified as independent primary tumours.

N – Regional Lymph Nodes

NX   Regional lymph nodes cannot be assessed
N0   No regional lymph node metastasis
N1   Regional lymph node metastasis

M – Distant Metastasis

M0   No distant metastasis
M1   Distant metastasis (excluding adnexa, pelvic and abdominal tissues)

pTNM Pathological Classification

The pT and pN categories correspond to the T and N categories. For pM see page 15.

Stage Grouping
(Uterine sarcomas)

Stage I	T1	N0	M0
Stage IA	T1a	N0	M0
Stage IB	T1b	N0	M0
Stage IC*	T1c	N0	M0
Stage II	T2	N0	M0
Stage IIA	T2a	N0	M0
Stage IIB	T2b	N0	M0
Stage IIIA	T3a	N0	M0
Stage IIIB	T3b	N0	M0
Stage IIIC	T1, T2, T3	N1	M0
Stage IVA	T4	Any N	M0
Stage IVB	Any T	Any N	M1

Note: * Stage IC does not apply for leiomyosarcoma and endometrial stromal sarcoma.

Summary

T1	Uterus
T2	Within pelvis
T3	Abdominal tissues
T4	Bladder/rectal mucosa

Ovary
(ICD-O C56)

The definitions of the T, N, and M categories correspond to the FIGO stages. Both systems are included for comparison.

Rules for Classification

The classification applies to malignant ovarian neoplasms of both epithelial and stromal origin including those of borderline malignancy or of low malignant potential (*WHO Classification of Tumours. Pathology and Genetics. Tumours of the Breast and Female Genital Organs*. Tavassoli FA, Devilee P eds. Geneva: WHO; 2003) corresponding to 'common epithelial tumours' of the earlier terminology.

There should be histological confirmation of the disease and division of cases by histological type.

The following are the procedures for assessing T, N, and M categories:

T categories	Clinical examination, imaging, surgical exploration (laparoscopy/laparotomy)
N categories	Clinical examination, imaging, surgical exploration (laparoscopy/laparotomy)
M categories	Clinical examination, imaging, surgical exploration (laparoscopy/laparotomy)

The FIGO stages are based on surgical staging. (TNM stages are based on clinical and/or pathological classification).

Regional Lymph Nodes

The regional lymph nodes are the hypogastric (including obturator), common iliac, external iliac, lateral sacral, para-aortic, and inguinal nodes.

TNM Clinical Classification

T – Primary Tumour

TNM Categories	FIGO Stages	
TX		Primary tumour cannot be assessed
T0		No evidence of primary tumour
T1	I	Tumour limited to the ovaries (one or both)
T1a	IA	Tumour limited to one ovary; capsule intact, no tumour on ovarian surface; no malignant cells in ascites or peritoneal washings
T1b	IB	Tumour limited to both ovaries; capsule intact, no tumour on ovarian surface; no malignant cells in ascites or peritoneal washings neal washings
T1c	IC	Tumour limited to one or both ovaries with any of the

		following: capsule ruptured, tumour on ovarian surface, malignant cells in ascites or peritoneal washings
T2	II	Tumour involves one or both ovaries with pelvic extension
T2a	IIA	Extension and/or implants on uterus and/or tube(s); no malignant cells in ascites or peritoneal washings
T2b	IIB	Extension to other pelvic tissues; no malignant cells in ascites or peritoneal washings
T2c	IIC	Pelvic extension (2a or 2b) with malignant cells in ascites or peritoneal washings
T3 and/ or N1	III	Tumour involves one or both ovaries with microscopically confirmed pertoneal metastasis outside the pelvis and/or regional lymph node metastasis
T3a	IIIA	Microscopic peritoneal metastasis beyond pelvis
T3b	IIIB	Macroscopic peritoneal, metastasis beyond pelvis, 2 cm or less in greatest dimension
T3c and/ or N1	IIIC	Peritoneal metastasis beyond pelvis, more than 2 cm in greatest dimension and/or regional lymph node metastasis
M1	IV	Distant metastasis (excludes peritoneal metastasis)

Note: Liver capsule metastasis is T3/Stage III, liver parenchymal metastasis M1/Stage IV. Pleural effusion must have positive cytology for M1/Stage IV.

N – Regional Lymph Nodes

NX   Regional lymph nodes cannot be assessed

N0   No regional lymph node metastasis

N1   Regional lymph node metastasis

M – Distant Metastasis

M0   No distant metastasis

M1   Distant metastasis except peritoneal metastasis

pTNM Pathological Classification

The pT and pN categories correspond to the T and N categories. For pM see page 15.

pN0   Histological examination of a pelvic lymphadenectomy specimen will ordinarily include 6 or more lymph nodes.

If the lymph nodes are negative, but the number ordinarily examined is not met, classify as pN0. (FIGO considers such cases as pNX)

G Histopathological Grading

See definitions on page 195.

Stage Grouping

Stage IA	T1a	N0	M0
Stage IB	T1b	N0	M0
Stage IC	T1c	N0	M0
Stage IIA	T2a	N0	M0
Stage IIB	T2b	N0	M0
Stage IIC	T2c	N0	M0
Stage IIIA	T3a	N0	M0
Stage IIIB	T3b	N0	M0
Stage IIIC	T3c	N0	M0
	Any T	N1	M0
Stage IV	Any T	Any N	M1

Summary

TNM	Ovary	FIGO
T1	Limited to the ovaries	I
T1a	One ovary, capsule intact	IA
T1b	Both ovaries, capsule intact	IB
T1c	Capsule ruptured, tumour on surface, malignant cells in ascites or peritoneal washings	IC
T2	Pelvic extension	II
T2a	Uterus, tube(s)	IIA
T2b	Other pelvic tissues	IIB
T2c	Malignant cells in ascites or peritoneal washings	IIC
T3 and/ or N1	Peritoneal metastasis beyond pelvis and/or regional lymph node metastasis	III
T3a	Microscopic peritoneal metastasis	IIIA
T3b	Macroscopic peritoneal metastasis ≤2 cm	IIIB
T3c and/ or N1	Peritoneal metastasis >2 cm regional lymph node metastasis	IIIC
M1	Distant metastasis (excludes peritoneal metastasis)	IV

Fallopian Tube
(ICD-O C57.0)

The following classification for carcinoma of the fallopian tube is based on that of FIGO adopted in 1992. The definitions of the T, N, and M categories correspond to the FIGO stages. Both systems are included for comparison.

Rules for Classification

The classification applies only to carcinoma. There should be histological confirmation of the disease.

The following are the procedures for assessing T, N, and M categories:

T categories	Clinical examination, imaging, surgical exploration (laparoscopy/laparotomy)
N categories	Clinical examination, imaging, surgical exploration (laparoscopy/laparotomy)
M categories	Clinical examination, imaging, surgical exploration (laparoscopy/laparotomy)

The FIGO stages are based on surgico-pathological examination. (TNM stages are based on clinical and/or pathological staging.)

Regional Lymph Nodes

The regional lymph nodes are the hypogastric (internal iliac, obturator), common iliac, external iliac, lateral sacral, para-aortic, and inguinal nodes.

TNM Clinical Classification

T – Primary Tumour

TNM Categories	FIGO Stages	
TX		Primary tumour cannot be assessed
T0		No evidence of primary tumour
Tis	*	Carcinoma in situ (preinvasive carcinoma)
T1	I	Tumour confined to fallopian tube(s)
T1a	IA	Tumour limited to one tube, without penetrating the serosal surface
T1b	IB	Tumour limited to both tubes, without penetrating the serosal surface
T1c	IC	Tumour limited to one or both tube(s) with extension onto or through the tubal serosa, or with malignant cells in ascites or peritoneal washings
T2	II	Tumour involves one or both fallopian tube(s) with pelvic extension

T2a	IIA	Extension and/or metastasis to uterus and/or ovaries
T2b	IIB	Extension to other pelvic structures
T2c	IIC	Pelvic extension (2a or 2b) with malignant cells in ascites or peritoneal washings
T3 and/or N1	III	Tumour involves one or both fallopian tube(s) with peritoneal implants outside the pelvis and/or positive regional lymph nodes
T3a	IIIA	Microscopic peritoneal metastasis outside the pelvis
T3b	IIIB	Macroscopic peritoneal metastasis outside the pelvis, 2 cm or less in greatest dimension
T3c and/ or N1	IIIC	Peritoneal metastasis, more than 2 cm in greatest dimension and/or positive regional lymph nodes
M1	IV	Distant metastasis (excludes peritoneal metastasis)

Note: Liver capsule metastasis is T3/Stage III, liver parenchymal metastasis, M1/Stage IV. Pleural effusion must have positive cytology for M1/Stage IV.

*FIGO no longer includes Stage 0 (Tis).

N – Regional Lymph nodes

NX   Regional lymph nodes cannot be assessed
N0   No regional lymph node metastasis
N1   Regional lymph node metastasis

M – Distant Metastasis

M0   No distant metastasis
M1   Distant metastasis

pTNM Pathological Classification

The pT and pN categories correspond to the T and N categories. For pM see page 15.

pN0   Histological examination of a pelvic lymphadenectomy specimen will ordinarily include 6 or more lymph nodes.

If the examined lymph nodes are negative, but the number ordinarily examined is not met, classify as pN0. (FIGO considers such cases as pNX).

G Histopathological Grading

See definitions on page 195.

Stage Grouping

Stage 0	Tis	N0	M0
Stage IA	T1a	N0	M0
Stage IB	T1b	N0	M0
Stage IC	T1c	N0	M0
Stage IIA	T2a	N0	M0
Stage IIB	T2b	N0	M0
Stage IIC	T2c	N0	M0
Stage IIIA	T3a	N0	M0
Stage IIIB	T3b	N0	M0
Stage IIIC	T3c	N0	M0
	Any T	N1	M0
Stage IV	Any T	Any N	M1

Summary

TNM	Fallopian Tube	FIGO
Tis	Carcinoma in situ	
T1	Limited to tube(s)	I
T1a	One tube; serosa intact	IA
T1b	Both tubes; serosa intact	IB
T1c	Serosa involved; malignant cells in ascites or peritoneal washings	IC
T2	Pelvic extension	II
T2a	Uterus and/or ovaries	IIA
T2b	Other pelvic structures	IIB
T2c	Malignant cells in ascites or peritoneal washings	IIC
T3 and/ or N1	Peritoneal metastasis outside the pelvis and/or regional lymph node metastasis	III
T3a	Microscopic peritoneal metastasis	IIIA
T3b	Macroscopic peritoneal metastasis ≤2 cm	IIIB
T3c and/ or N1	Peritoneal metastasis >2 cm and/or regional lymph node metastasis	IIIC
M1	Distant metastasis (excludes peritoneal metastasis)	IV

Gestational Trophoblastic Tumours
(ICD-O C58)

The following classification for gestational trophoblastic tumours is based on that of FIGO adopted in 1992 and updated in 2002 (Ngan HYS, Bender H, Benedet JL, et al. [FIGO Committee on Gynecologic Oncology]. Gestational trophoblastic neoplasia. *Int J Gynecol Obstet* 2002; 77:285–287). The definitions of T and M categories correspond to the FIGO stages. Both systems are included for comparison. In contrast to other sites, an N (regional lymph node) classification does not apply to these tumours. A prognostic scoring index, which is based on factors other than the anatomic extent of the disease, is used to assign cases to high risk and low risk categories, and these categories are used in stage grouping.

Rules for Classification

The classification applies to choriocarcinoma (9100/3), invasive hydatidiform mole (9100/1), and placental site trophoblastic tumour (9104/1). Placental site tumours should be reported separately. Histological confirmation is not required if the human chorionic gonadotropin (ßhCG) level is abnormally elevated. History of prior chemotherapy for this disease should be noted.

The following are the procedures for assessing T and M categories:

T categories:	Clinical examination, imaging and endoscopy, and serum/urine βhCG level
M categories:	Clinical examination, imaging, and assessment of serum/urine βhCG level
Risk categories:	Age, type of antecedent pregnancy, interval months from index pregnancy, pretreatment serum/urine βhCG, diameter of largest tumour, site of metastasis, number of metastases, and previous failed chemotherapy are integrated to provide a prognostic score that divides cases into low and high risk categories.

TM Clinical Classification

T– Primary Tumour

TM Categories	FIGO Stages*	
TX		Primary tumour cannot be assessed
T0		No evidence of primary tumour
T1	I	Tumour confined to uterus

T2	II	Tumour extends to other genital structures: vagina, ovary, broad ligament, fallopian tube by metastasis or direct extension
M1a	III	Metastasis to lung(s)
M1b	IV	Other distant metastasis

Note: *Stages I–IV are subdivided into A and B according to the prognostic score.

M – Distant Metastasis

M0	No distant metastasis
M1	Distant metastasis
M1a	Metastasis to lung(s)
M1b	Other distant metastasis

Note: Genital metastasis (vagina, ovary, broad ligament, fallopian tube) is classified T2. Any involvement of non-genital structures, whether by direct invasion or metastasis is described using the M classification.

pTM Pathological Classification

The pT categories correspond to the T categories. For pM see page 15.

Prognostic Score

Prognostic Factor	0	1	2	4
Age	<40	≥40		
Antecedent pregnancy	H. mole	Abortion	Term pregnancy	
Months from index pregnancy	<4	4–6	7–12	>12
Pretreatment Serum βhCG (IU/ml)	$<10^3$	$10^3–<10^4$	$10^4–<10^5$	$≥10^5$
Largest tumour size including uterus	<3 cm	3–5 cm	>5 cm	
Sites of metastasis	Lung	Spleen, kidney	Gastrointestinal tract	Liver, brain
Number of metastasis		1–4	5–8	>8
Previous failed chemotherapy			Single drug	Two or more drugs

Risk Categories
Total prognostic score 6 or less = low risk
Total score 7 or more = high risk

Prognostic Grouping

Group	T	M	Risk Category
I	T1	M0	Unknown
IA	T1	M0	Low
IB	T1	M0	High
II	T2	M0	Unknown
IIA	T2	M0	Low
IIB	T2	M0	High
III	Any T	M1a	Unknown
IIIA	Any T	M1a	Low
IIIB	Any T	M1a	High
IV	Any T	M1b	Unknown
IVA	Any T	M1b	Low
IVB	Any T	M1b	High

Summary

TM and risk	Gestational Trophoblastic Tumours	Stage
T1	Confined to uterus	I
T2	Other genital structures	II
M1a	Metastasis to lung(s)	III
M1b	Other distant metastasis	IV
Low risk	Prognostic score 6 or less	IA–IVA
High risk	Prognostic score 7 or more	IB–IVB

UROLOGICAL TUMOURS

Introductory Notes

The following sites are included:

- Penis
- Prostate
- Testis
- Kidney
- Renal pelvis and ureter
- Urinary bladder
- Urethra

Each site is described under the following headings:

- Rules for classification with the procedures for assessing T, N, and M categories; additional methods may be used when they enhance the accuracy of appraisal before treatment
- Anatomical sites and subsites where appropriate
- Definition of the regional lymph nodes
- Distant metastasis
- TNM Clinical classification
- pTNM Pathological classification
- G Histopathological grading where applicable
- Stage grouping
- Summary

Distant Metastasis

The categories M1 and pM1 may be further specified according to the following notation:

Pulmonary	PUL	Bone marrow	MAR
Osseous	OSS	Pleura	PLE
Hepatic	HEP	Peritoneum	PER
Brain	BRA	Adrenals	ADR
Lymph nodes	LYM	Skin	SKI
Others	OTH		

R Classification

See Introduction, page 19.

Penis
(ICD-O C60)

Rules for Classification

The classification applies to carcinomas. There should be histological confirmation of the disease.
The following are the procedures for assessing T, N, and M categories:

T categories	Physical examination and endoscopy
N categories	Physical examination and imaging
M categories	Physical examination and imaging

Anatomical Subsites

1. Prepuce (C60.0)
2. Glans penis (C60.1)
3. Body of penis (C60.2)

Regional Lymph Nodes

The regional lymph nodes are the superficial and deep inguinal and the pelvic nodes.

TNM Clinical Classification

T – Primary Tumour

TX   Primary tumour cannot be assessed
T0   No evidence of primary tumour
Tis   Carcinoma in situ
Ta   Non-invasive verrucous carcinoma[1]

T1   Tumour invades subepithelial connective tissue
    T1a   Tumour invades subepithelial connective tissue without lymphovascular invasion and is not poorly differentiated or undifferentiated
    T1b   Tumour invades subepithelial connective tissue with lymphovascular invasion or is poorly differentiated or undifferentiated
T2   Tumour invades corpus spongiosum or cavernosum
T3   Tumour invades urethra
T4   Tumour invades other adjacent structures

Note: 1. Verrucous carcinoma not associated with destructive invasion.

N – Regional Lymph Nodes

NX   Regional lymph nodes cannot be assessed
N0   No palpable or visibly enlarged inguinal lymph nodes
N1   Palpable mobile unilateral inguinal lymph node
N2   Palpable mobile multiple or bilateral inguinal lymph nodes
N3   Fixed inguinal nodal mass or pelvic lymphadenopathy unilateral or bilateral

M – Distant Metastasis

M0   No distant metastasis
M1   Distant metastasis

pTNM Pathological Classification

The pT categories correspond to the T categories. The pN categories are based upon biopsy, or surgical excision. For pM see page 15.

pNX   Regional lymph nodes cannot be assessed
pN0   No regional lymph node metastasis
pN1   Metastasis in a single inguinal lymph node
pN2   Metastasis in multiple or bilateral inguinal lymph nodes
pN3   Metastasis in pelvic lymph node(s), unilateral or bilateral or extranodal extension of regional lymph node metastasis

G Histopathological Grading

GX   Grade of differentiation cannot be assessed
G1   Well differentiated
G2   Moderately differentiated
G3–4   Poorly differentiated/undifferentiated

Stage Grouping

Stage 0	Tis	N0	M0
	Ta	N0	M0
Stage I	T1a	N0	M0
Stage II	T1b	N0	M0
	T2	N0, N1	M0
	T3	N0	M0
Stage IIIA	T1, T2, T3	N1	M0
Stage IIIB	T1, T2, T3	N2	M0
Stage IV	T4	Any N	M0
	Any T	N3	M0
	Any T	Any N	M1

Summary

Penis			
Tis	Carcinoma in situ		
Ta	Non-invasive verrucous carcinoma		
T1	Subepithelial connective tissue		
T2	Corpus spongiosum, cavernosum		
T3	Urethra		
T4	Other adjacent structures		
N1	Single palpable mobile unilateral inguinal	pN1	Single inguinal
N2	Palpable mobile multiple or bilateral inguinal	pN2	Multiple/bilateral inguinal
N3	Fixed inguinal or pelvic	pN3	Pelvic or extranodal

Prostate
(ICD-O C61)

Rules for Classification

The classification applies only to adenocarcinomas. Transitional cell carcinoma of the prostate is classified as a urethral tumour (see page 266). There should be histological confirmation of the disease.

The following are the procedures for assessing T, N, and M categories:

T categories	Physical examination, imaging, endoscopy, biopsy, and biochemical tests
N categories	Physical examination and imaging
M categories	Physical examination, imaging, skeletal studies, and biochemical tests

Regional Lymph Nodes

The regional lymph nodes are the nodes of the true pelvis, which essentially are the pelvic nodes below the bifurcation of the common iliac arteries. Laterality does not affect the N classification.

TNM Clinical Classification

T – Primary Tumour

TX   Primary tumour cannot be assessed
T0   No evidence of primary tumour

T1   Clinically inapparent tumour, neither palpable nor visible by imaging

    T1a   Tumour incidental histological finding in 5% or less of tissue resected

    T1b   Tumour incidental histological finding in more than 5% of tissue resected

    T1c   Tumour identified by needle biopsy, e.g., because of elevated prostate-specific antigen (PSA)

T2   Tumour confined within prostate[1]

    T2a   Tumour involves one-half of one lobe or less

    T2b   Tumour involves more than one-half of one lobe, but not both lobes

    T2c   Tumour involves both lobes

T3   Tumour extends through the prostatic capsule[2]

    T3a   Extracapsular extension (unilateral or bilateral) including microscopic bladder neck involvement

    T3b   Tumour invades seminal vesicle(s)

T4   Tumour is fixed or invades adjacent structures other than seminal vesicles: external sphincter, rectum, levator muscles, and/or pelvic wall

Notes: 1. Tumour found in one or both lobes by needle biopsy, but not palpable or reliably visible by imaging, is classified as T1c.

       2. Invasion into the prostatic apex or into (but not beyond) the prostatic capsule is not classified as T3, but as T2.

N – Regional Lymph Nodes

NX   Regional lymph nodes cannot be assessed

N0   No regional lymph node metastasis

N1   Regional lymph node metastasis

M – Distant Metastasis*

M0   No distant metastasis

M1   Distant metastasis

      M1a Non-regional lymph node(s)

      M1b Bone(s)

      M1c Other site(s)

Note: *When more than one site of metastasis is present, the most advanced category is used. pM1c is the most advanced category.

pTNM Pathological Classification

The pT and pN categories correspond to the T and N categories. For pM see page 15.

However, there is no pT1 category because there is insufficient tissue to assess the highest pT category.

Note: Metastasis no larger than 0.2 cm can be designated pN1 mi. (see Introduction, pN, page 13.)

G Histopathological Grading

GX   Grade cannot be assessed

G1   Well differentiated (slight anaplasia) (Gleason 2–4)

G2   Moderately differentiated (moderate anaplasia) (Gleason 5–6)

G3–4 Poorly differentiated/undifferentiated (marked anaplasia) (Gleason 7–10)

Stage Grouping

Stage I	T1, T2a	N0	M0
Stage II	T2b, T2c	N0	M0
Stage III	T3	N0	M0
Stage IV	T4	N0	M0
	Any T	N1	M0
	Any T	Any N	M1

Prognostic Grouping

Group I	T1a–c	N0	M0	PSA <10	Gleason ≤6
	T2a	N0	M0	PSA <10	Gleason ≤6
Group IIA	T1a–c	N0	M0	PSA < 20	Gleason 7
	T1a–c	N0	M0	PSA ≥10<20	Gleason ≤6
	T2a, b	N0	M0	PSA <20	Gleason ≤7
Group IIB	T2c	N0	M0	Any PSA	Any Gleason
	T1–2	N0	M0	PSA ≥20	Any Gleason
	T1–2	N0	M0	Any PSA	Gleason ≥8
Group III	T3a, b	N0	M0	Any PSA	Any Gleason
Group IV	T4	N0	M0	Any PSA	Any Gleason
	Any T	N1	M0	Any PSA	Any Gleason
	Any T	Any N	M1	Any PSA	Any Gleason

Note: When either PSA or Gleason is not available, grouping should be determined by T category and whichever of either PSA or Gleason is available. When neither is available prognostic grouping is not possible, use stage grouping

Summary

Prostate	
T1	Not palpable or visible
T1a	≤5%
T1b	>5%
T1c	Needle biopsy
T2	Confined within prostate
T2a	≤ One-half of one lobe
T2b	More than one-half of one lobe
T2c	Both lobes
T3	Through prostatic capsule
T3a	Extracapsular
T3b	Seminal vesicle(s)
T4	Fixed or invades adjacent structures: external sphincter, rectum, levator muscles, pelvic wall
N1	Regional lymph node(s)
M1a	Non-regional lymph node(s)
M1b	Bone(s)
M1c	Other site(s)

Testis
(ICD-O C62)

Rules for Classification

The classification applies to germ cell tumours of the testis. There should be histological confirmation of the disease and division of cases by histological type. Histopathological grading is not applicable.

The presence of elevated serum tumour markers, including alphafetoprotein (AFP), hCG and LDH, is frequent in this disease. Staging is based on the determination of the anatomic extent of disease and assessment of serum tumour markers.

The following are the procedures for assessing N, M, and S categories:

N categories	Physical examination and imaging
M categories	Physical examination, imaging, and biochemical tests
S categories	Serum tumour markers

Serum tumour markers are obtained immediately after orchiectomy and, if elevated, should be performed serially after orchiectomy according to the normal decay for AFP (half-life 7 days) and βhCG (half-life 3 days) to assess for serum tumour marker elevation. The S classification is based on the nadir value of hCG and AFP after orchiectomy. The serum level of LDH (but not its half-life levels) has prognostic value in patients with metastatic disease and is included for staging.

Regional Lymph Nodes

The regional lymph nodes are the abdominal para-aortic (periaortic), preaortic, interaortocaval, precaval, paracaval, retrocaval, and retroaortic nodes. Nodes along the spermatic vein should be considered regional. Laterality does not affect the N classification. The intrapelvic nodes and the inguinal nodes are considered regional after scrotal or inguinal surgery.

TNM Clinical Classification

T – Primary Tumour

Except for pT4, where radical orchiectomy is not always necessary for classification purposes, the extent of the primary tumour is classified after radical orchiectomy; see pT. In other circumstances, TX is used if no radical orchiectomy has been performed.

N – Regional Lymph Nodes

NX   Regional lymph nodes cannot be assessed

N0   No regional lymph node metastasis

N1   Metastasis with a lymph node mass 2 cm or less in greatest dimension or multiple lymph nodes, none more than 2 cm in greatest dimension

N2 Metastasis with a lymph node mass more than 2 cm but not more than 5 cm in greatest dimension, or multiple lymph nodes, any one mass more than 2 cm but not more than 5 cm in greatest dimension

N3 Metastasis with a lymph node mass more than 5 cm in greatest dimension

M – Distant Metastasis

M0 No distant metastasis
M1 Distant metastasis
  M1a Non-regional lymph node(s) or lung metastasis
  M1b Distant metastasis other than non-regional lymph nodes and lung

pTNM Pathological Classification

pT – Primary Tumour

pTX Primary tumour cannot be assessed (see T – Primary Tumour, above)

pT0 No evidence of primary tumour (e.g., histological scar in testis)

pTis Intratubular germ cell neoplasia (carcinoma in situ)

pT1 Tumour limited to testis and epididymis without vascular/lymphatic invasion; tumour may invade tunica albuginea but not tunica vaginalis

pT2 Tumour limited to testis and epididymis with vascular/lymphatic invasion, or tumour extending through tunica albuginea with involvement of tunica vaginalis

pT3 Tumour invades spermatic cord with or without vascular/lymphatic invasion

pT4 Tumour invades scrotum with or without vascular/lymphatic invasion

pN – Regional Lymph Nodes

pNX   Regional lymph nodes cannot be assessed
pN0   No regional lymph node metastasis
pN1   Metastasis with a lymph node mass 2 cm or less in greatest dimension or 5 or fewer positive nodes, none more than 2 cm in greatest dimension
pN2   Metastasis with a lymph node mass more than 2 cm but not more than 5 cm in greatest dimension; or more than 5 nodes positive, none more than 5 cm; or evidence of extranodal extension of tumour
pN3   Metastasis with a lymph node mass more than 5 cm in greatest dimension

pM – Distant Metastasis

For pM see page 15.

S – Serum Tumour Markers

	LDH	βhCG (mIU/ml)	AFP (ng/ml)
SX	Serum marker studies not available		
S0	Serum marker study levels within normal limits		
S1	$<1.5 \times N$	and <5000	and <1000
S2	$1.5–10 \times N$	or $5000–50\,000$	or $1000–10\,000$
S3	$>10 \times N$	or $>50\,000$	or $>10\,000$

Note: N indicates the upper limit of normal for the LDH assay.

Stage grouping

Stage 0	pTis	N0	M0	S0, SX
Stage I	pT1 – T4	N0	M0	SX
Stage IA	pT1	N0	M0	S0
Stage IB	pT2 – T4	N0	M0	S0
Stage IS	Any pT/TX	N0	M0	S1 – S3
Stage II	Any pT/TX	N1 – N3	M0	SX
Stage IIA	Any pT/TX	N1	M0	S0
	Any pT/TX	N1	M0	S1
Stage IIB	Any pT/TX	N2	M0	S0
	Any pT/TX	N2	M0	S1
Stage IIC	Any pT/TX	N3	M0	S0
	Any pT/TX	N3	M0	S1
Stage III	Any pT/TX	Any N	M1a	SX
Stage IIIA	Any pT/TX	Any N	M1a	S0
	Any pT/TX	Any N	M1a	S1
Stage IIIB	Any pT/TX	N1 – N3	M0	S2
	Any pT/TX	Any N	M1a	S2
Stage IIIC	Any pT/TX	N1 – N3	M0	S3
	Any pT/TX	Any N	M1a	S3
	Any pT/TX	Any N	M1b	Any S

Summary

Testis			
pTis	Intratubular		
pT1	Testis and epididymis, no vascular/lymphatic invasion		
pT2	Testis and epididymis with vascular/lymphatic invasion or tunica vaginalis		
pT3	Spermatic cord		
pT4	Scrotum		
N1	≤2 cm	pN1	≤2 cm and ≤5 nodes
N2	>2 cm to 5 cm	pN2	>2 cm to 5 cm or >5 nodes or extranodal extension
N3	>5 cm	pN3	>5 cm
M1a	Non-regional lymph nodes or lung		
M1b	Other sites		

Kidney
(ICD-O C64)

Rules for Classification

The classification applies to renal cell carcinoma. There should be histological confirmation of the disease.

The following are the procedures for assessing T, N, and M categories:

T categories	Physical examination and imaging
N categories	Physical examination and imaging
M categories	Physical examination and imaging

Regional Lymph Nodes

The regional lymph nodes are the hilar, abdominal para-aortic, and paracaval nodes. Laterality does not affect the N categories.

TNM Clinical Classification

T – Primary Tumour

TX   Primary tumour cannot be assessed
T0   No evidence of primary tumour

T1   Tumour 7 cm or less in greatest dimension, limited to the kidney
  T1a Tumour 4 cm or less
  T1b Tumour more than 4 cm but not more than 7 cm

T2 Tumour more than 7 cm in greatest dimension, limited to the kidney

  T2a Tumour more than 7 cm but not more than 10 cm

  T2b Tumour more than 10 cm, limited to the kidney

T3 Tumour extends into major veins or perinephric tissues but not into the ipsilateral adrenal gland and not beyond Gerota fascia

  T3a Tumour grossly extends into the renal vein or its segmental (muscle containing) branches, or tumour invades perirenal and/or renal sinus fat (peripelvic) fat but not beyond Gerota fascia

  T3b Tumour grossly extends into vena cava below diaphragm

  T3c Tumour grossly extends into vena cava above the diaphragm or invades the wall of the vena cava

T4 Tumour invades beyond Gerota fascia (including contiguous extension into the ipsilateral adrenal gland)

N – Regional Lymph Nodes

NX Regional lymph nodes cannot be assessed
N0 No regional lymph node metastasis
N1 Metastasis in a single regional lymph node
N2 Metastasis in more than one regional lymph node

M – Distant Metastasis

M0 No distant metastasis
M1 Distant metastasis

pTNM Pathological Classification

The pT and pN categories correspond to the T and N categories. For pM see page 15.

G Histopathological Grading

GX   Grade of differentiation cannot be assessed
G1   Well differentiated
G2   Moderately differentiated
G3–4 Poorly differentiated/undifferentiated

Stage Grouping

Stage I	T1	N0	M0
Stage II	T2	N0	M0
Stage III	T3	N0	M0
	T1, T2, T3	N1	M0
Stage IV	T4	Any N	M0
	Any T	N2	M0
	Any T	Any N	M1

Summary

Kidney

T1	≤7 cm; limited to the kidney
T1a	≤4 cm
T1b	>4 cm
T2	>7 cm; limited to the kidney
T2a	>7 to 10 cm
T2b	>10 cm
T3	major veins, perinephric fat
T3a	Renal vein, perinephric fat
T3b	Vena cava below diaphragm
T3c	Vena cava above diaphragm
T4	Beyond Gerota fascia, ipsilateral adrenal
N1	Single
N2	More than one

Renal Pelvis and Ureter
(ICD-O C65, C66)

Rules for Classification

The classification applies to carcinomas. Papilloma is excluded. There should be histological or cytological confirmation of the disease.

The following are the procedures for assessing T, N, and M categories:

T categories	Physical examination, imaging, and endoscopy
N categories	Physical examination and imaging
M categories	Physical examination and imaging

Anatomical Sites

1. Renal pelvis (C65)
2. Ureter (C66)

Regional Lymph Nodes

The regional lymph nodes are the hilar, abdominal para-aortic, and paracaval nodes and, for ureter, intrapelvic nodes. Laterality does not affect the N classification.

TNM Clinical Classification

T – Primary Tumour

TX	Primary tumour cannot be assessed
T0	No evidence of primary tumour
Ta	Non-invasive papillary carcinoma
Tis	Carcinoma in situ

T1	Tumour invades subepithelial connective tissue
T2	Tumour invades muscularis
T3	*(Renal pelvis)* Tumour invades beyond muscularis into peripelvic fat or renal parenchyma *(Ureter)* Tumour invades beyond muscularis into periureteric fat
T4	Tumour invades adjacent organs or through the kidney into perinephric fat

N – Regional Lymph Nodes

NX	Regional lymph nodes cannot be assessed
N0	No regional lymph node metastasis
N1	Metastasis in a single lymph node 2 cm or less in greatest dimension
N2	Metastasis in a single lymph node more than 2 cm but not more than 5 cm in greatest dimension, or multiple lymph nodes, none more than 5 cm in greatest dimension
N3	Metastasis in a lymph node more than 5 cm in greatest dimension

M – Distant Metastasis

M0	No distant metastasis
M1	Distant metastasis

pTNM Pathological Classification

The pT and pN categories correspond to the T and N categories. For pM see page 15.

G Histopathological Grading

GX   Grade of differentiation cannot be assessed
G1   Well differentiated
G2   Moderately differentiated
G3–4   Poorly differentiated/undifferentiated

Stage Grouping

Stage 0a	Ta	N0	M0
Stage 0is	Tis	N0	M0
Stage I	T1	N0	M0
Stage II	T2	N0	M0
Stage III	T3	N0	M0
Stage IV	T4	N0	M0
	Any T	N1, N2, N3	M0
	Any T	Any N	M1

Summary

Renal Pelvis, Ureter

Ta	Non-invasive papillary
Tis	In situ
T1	Subepithelial connective tissue
T2	Muscularis
T3	Beyond muscularis
T4	Adjacent organs, perinephric fat
N1	Single ≤2 cm
N2	Single >2 cm to 5 cm, multiple ≤5 cm
N3	>5 cm

Urinary Bladder
(ICD-O C67)

Rules for Classification

The classification applies to carcinomas. Papilloma is excluded. There should be histological or cytological confirmation of the disease.

The following are the procedures for assessing T, N, and M categories:

T categories	Physical examination, imaging, and endoscopy
N categories	Physical examination and imaging
M categories	Physical examination and imaging

Regional Lymph Nodes

The regional lymph nodes are the nodes of the true pelvis, which essentially are the pelvic nodes below the bifurcation of the common iliac arteries, but include the lymph nodes along the common iliac artery too. Laterality does not affect the N classification.

TNM Clinical Classification

T – Primary Tumour

The suffix (m) should be added to the appropriate T category to indicate multiple tumours. The suffix (is) may be added to any T to indicate presence of associated carcinoma in situ.

TX   Primary tumour cannot be assessed
T0   No evidence of primary tumour
Ta   Non-invasive papillary carcinoma
Tis   Carcinoma in situ: 'flat tumour'

T1   Tumour invades subepithelial connective tissue
T2   Tumour invades muscle

    T2a   Tumour invades superficial muscle (inner half)

    T2b   Tumour invades deep muscle (outer half)

T3   Tumour invades perivesical tissue:

    T3a   microscopically

    T3b   macroscopically (extravesical mass)

T4   Tumour invades any of the following: prostate stroma, seminal vesicles, uterus, vagina, pelvic wall, abdominal wall

    T4a   Tumour invades prostate stroma, seminal vesicles, uterus, or vagina

    T4b   Tumour invades pelvic wall or abdominal wall

N – Regional Lymph Nodes

NX   Regional lymph nodes cannot be assessed
N0   No regional lymph node metastasis
N1   Metastasis in a single lymph node in the true pelvis (hypogastric, obturator, external iliac, or presacral)
N2   Metastasis in multiple lymph nodes in the true pelvis (hypogastric, obturator, external iliac, or presacral)
N3   Metastasis in a common iliac lymph node(s)

M – Distant Metastasis

M0   No distant metastasis
M1   Distant metastasis

pTNM Pathological Classification

The pT and pN categories correspond to the T and N categories. For pM see page 15.

G Histopathological Grading

GX   Grade of differentiation cannot be assessed
G1   Well differentiated
G2   Moderately differentiated
G3–4 Poorly differentiated/undifferentiated

Stage Grouping

Stage 0a	Ta	N0	M0
Stage 0is	Tis	N0	M0
Stage I	T1	N0	M0
Stage II	T2a, b	N0	M0
Stage III	T3a, b	N0	M0
	T4a	N0	M0
Stage IV	T4b	N0	M0
	Any T	N1, N2, N3	M0
	Any T	Any N	M1

Summary

Urinary Bladder	
Ta	Non-invasive papillary
Tis	In situ: 'flat tumour'
T1	Subepithelial connective tissue
T2	Muscularis
T2a	Inner half
T2b	Outer half
T3	Beyond muscularis
T3a	Microscopically
T3b	Extravesical mass
T4	Prostate, uterus, vagina, pelvic wall, abdominal wall
T4a	Prostate, uterus, vagina
T4b	Pelvic wall, abdominal wall
N1	Single
N2	Multiple
N3	Common iliac

Urethra
(ICD 0 (68.0, C61.9))

Rules for Classification

The classification applies to carcinomas of the urethra (ICD-O C68.0) and transitional cell carcinomas of the prostate (ICD-O C61.9) and prostatic urethra. There should be histological or cytological confirmation of the disease.

The following are the procedures for assessing T, N, and M categories:

T categories	Physical examination, imaging, and endoscopy
N categories	Physical examination and imaging
M categories	Physical examination and imaging

Regional Lymph Nodes

The regional lymph nodes are the inguinal and the pelvic nodes. Laterality does not affect the N classification.

TNM Clinical Classification

T – Primary Tumour

TX   Primary tumour cannot be assessed
T0   No evidence of primary tumour

Urethra (male and female)

Ta   Non-invasive papillary, polypoid, or verrucous carcinoma
Tis   Carcinoma in situ

T1   Tumour invades subepithelial connective tissue
T2   Tumour invades any of the following: corpus spongiosum, prostate, periurethral muscle
T3   Tumour invades any of the following: corpus cavernosum, beyond prostatic capsule, bladder neck (extraprostatic extension)
T4   Tumour invades other adjacent organs (invasion of the bladder)

Urothelial (Transitional cell) carcinoma of the prostate

Tis pu Carcinoma in situ, involvement of prostatic urethra
Tis pd Carcinoma in situ, involvement of prostatic ducts

T1   Tumour invades subepithelial connective tissue (for tumours involving prostatic urethra only)
T2   Tumour invades any of the following: prostatic stroma, corpus spongiosum, periurethral muscle
T3   Tumour invades any of the following: corpus cavernosum, beyond prostatic capsule, bladder neck (extraprostatic extension)
T4   Tumour invades other adjacent organs (invasion of bladder)

N – Regional Lymph Nodes

NX   Regional lymph nodes cannot be assessed
N0   No regional lymph node metastasis
N1   Metastasis in a single lymph node 2 cm or less in greatest dimension
N2   Metastasis in a single lymph node more than 2 cm in greatest dimension, or in multiple lymph nodes

M – Distant Metastasis

M0   No distant metastasis
M1   Distant metastasis

pTNM Pathological Classification

The pT and pN categories correspond to the T and N categories. For pM see page 15.

G Histopathological Grading

GX   Grade of differentiation cannot be assessed
G1   Well differentiated
G2   Moderately differentiated
G3–4 Poorly differentiated/undifferentiated

Stage Grouping

Stage 0a	Ta	N0	M0
Stage 0is	Tis	N0	M0
	Tispu	N0	M0
	Tispd	N0	M0
Stage I	T1	N0	M0
Stage II	T2	N0	M0
Stage III	T1, T2	N1	M0
	T3	N0, N1	M0
Stage IV	T4	N0, N1	M0
	Any T	N2	M0
	Any T	Any N	M1

Summary

Urethra	
Ta	Non-invasive papillary, polypoid, or verrucous
Tis	In situ
T1	Subepithelial connective tissue
T2	Corpus spongiosum, prostate, periurethral muscle
T3	Corpus cavernosum, beyond prostatic capsule, anterior vagina, bladder neck
T4	Other adjacent organs

Urothelial (Transitional Cell) Carcinoma of Prostate (Prostatic Urethra)	
Tis pu	In situ, prostatic urethra
Tis pd	In situ, prostatic ducts
T1	Subepithelial connective tissue
T2	Prostatic stroma, corpus spongiosum, periurethral muscle
T3	Corpus cavernosum, beyond prostatic capsule, bladder neck (extraprostatic extension)
T4	Other adjacent organs (bladder)
N1	Single ≤2 cm
N2	>2 cm or multiple

ADRENAL CORTEX TUMOURS
(C74.0)

Rules for Classification

This classification applies to carcinomas of the adrenal cortex. It does not apply to tumours of the adrenal medulla or sarcomas.

The following are the procedures for assessing T, N, and M categories:

T categories	Physical examination and imaging
N categories	Physical examination and imaging
M categories	Physical examination and imaging

Regional Lymph Nodes

The regional lymph nodes are the hilar, abdominal para-aortic, and paracaval nodes. Laterality does not affect the N categories.

TNM Clinical Classification

T – Primary Tumour

TX   Primary tumour cannot be assessed
T0   No evidence of primary tumour

T1   Tumour 5 cm or less in greatest dimension, no extra-adrenal invasion

T2 Tumour greater than 5 cm, no extra-adrenal invasion

T3 Tumour of any size with local invasion, but not invading adjacent organs*

T4 Tumour of any size with invasion of adjacent organs*

Note: *Adjacent organs include kidney, diaphragm, great vessels, pancreas, and liver.

N – Regional lymph nodes

NX Regional lymph nodes cannot be assessed
N0 No regional lymph node metastasis
N1 Metastasis in regional lymph node(s)

M – Distant Metastasis

M0 No distance metastasis
M1 Distance metastasis

pTNM Pathological Classification

The pT and pN categories correspond to the T and N categories. For pM see page 15.

Stage Grouping

Stage I	T1	N0	M0
Stage II	T2	N0	M0
Stage III	T1, T2	N1	M0
	T3	N0	M0
Stage IV	T3	N1	M0
	T4	Any N	M0
	Any T	Any N	M1

Summary

Adrenal cortical carcinoma	
T1	≤5 cm, no extra-adrenal invasion
T2	>5 cm, no extra-adrenal invasion
T3	Local invasion
T4	Adjacent organs
N1	Regional

OPHTHALMIC TUMOURS

Introductory Notes

Tumours of the eye and its adnexa are a disparate group including carcinoma, melanoma, sarcomas, and retinoblastoma. For clinical convenience they are classified in one section.

The following sites are included:

- Conjunctiva
- Uvea
- Retina
- Orbit
- Lacrimal gland
- Eyelid (eyelid tumours are classified with skin tumours)

For histological nomenclature and diagnostic criteria, reference to the WHO histological classification (Campbell RJ. *Histological Typing of Tumours of the Eye and its Adnexa*, 2nd ed. Berlin: Springer; 1998) is recommended.

Each tumour type is described under the following headings:

- Rules for classification with the procedures for assessing the T, N, and M categories
- Anatomical sites where appropriate
- Definition of the regional lymph nodes
- TNM Clinical classification

- pTNM Pathological classification
- G Histopathological grading where applicable
- Stage grouping where applicable
- Summary

Regional Lymph Nodes

The definitions of N categories for ophthalmic tumours are:

N – Regional Lymph Nodes

NX   Regional lymph nodes cannot be assessed
N0   No regional lymph node metastasis
N1   Regional lymph node metastasis

Distant Metastasis

The definitions of the M categories for ophthalmic tumours are:

M — Distant Metastasis

M0   No distant metastasis
M1   Distant metastasis

The categories M1 and pM1 may be further specified according to the following notation:

Pulmonary	PUL	Bone marrow	MAR
Osseous	OSS	Pleura	PLE
Hepatic	HEP	Peritoneum	PER
Brain	BRA	Adrenals	ADR
Lymph nodes	LYM	Skin	SKI
Others	OTH		

G Histopathological Grading

The following definitions of the G categories apply to carcinoma of the conjunctiva and sarcoma of the orbit. These are:

GX   Grade of differentiation cannot be assessed
G1   Well differentiated
G2   Moderately differentiated
G3   Poorly differentiated
G4   Undifferentiated

R Classification

See Introduction, page 19.

Carcinoma of Conjunctiva
(ICD-O C69.0)

Rules for Classification

There should be histological confirmation of the disease and division of cases by histological type, e.g., mucoepidermoid and squamous cell carcinoma.

The following are the procedures for assessing T, N, and M categories:

T categories	Physical examination
N categories	Physical examination
M categories	Physical examination and imaging

Regional Lymph Nodes

The regional lymph nodes are the preauricular, submandibular and cervical lymph nodes.

TNM Clinical Classification

T – Primary Tumour

TX	Primary tumour cannot be assessed
T0	No evidence of primary tumour
Tis	Carcinoma in situ

T1   Tumour 5 mm or less in greatest dimension
T2   Tumour more than 5 mm in greatest dimension, without invasion of adjacent structures*
T3   Tumour invades adjacent structures*
T4   Tumour invades the orbit or beyond

>   T4a   Tumour invades orbital soft tissues, without bone invasion
>   T4b   Tumour invades bone
>   T4c   Tumour invades adjacent paranasal sinuses
>   T4d   Tumour invades brain

Notes: *Adjacent structures include: the cornea (3, 6, 9, or 12 clock hours), intraocular compartments, forniceal conjunctiva (lower and/or upper), palpebral conjunctiva (lower and/or upper), tarsal conjunctiva (lower and/or upper), lacrimal punctum and canaliculi (lower and/or upper), plica, caruncle, posterior eyelid lamella, anterior eyelid lamella, and/or eyelid margin (lower and/or upper).

N – Regional Lymph Nodes

NX   Regional lymph nodes cannot be assessed
N0   No regional lymph node metastasis
N1   Regional lymph node metastasis

M – Distant Metastasis

M0   No distant metastasis
M1   Distant metastasis

pTNM Pathological Classification

The pT and pN categories correspond to the T and N categories. For pM see page 15.

G Histopathological Grading

See definitions on page 275.

Stage Grouping

No stage grouping is at present recommended.

Summary

Conjunctiva Carcinoma	
T1	≤5 mm
T2	>5 mm
T3	Adjacent structures
T4	Orbit and beyond
N1	Regional

Malignant Melanoma of Conjunctiva
(ICD-O C69.0)

Rules for Classification

The classification applies to conjunctival malignant melanoma.

There should be histological confirmation of the disease.

The following are the procedures for assessing T, N, and M categories:

T categories	Physical examination
N categories	Physical examination
M categories	Physical examination and imaging

Regional Lymph Nodes

The regional lymph nodes are the preauricular, submandibular, and cervical lymph nodes.

TNM Clinical Classification

T – Primary Tumour

TX	Primary tumour cannot be assessed
T0	No evidence of primary tumour
Tis	Melanoma confined to the conjunctival epithelium (in situ)[1]

T1   Melanoma of the bulbar conjunctiva

    T1a   Tumour involves not more than one quadrant[2]

    T1b   Tumour involves more than one but not more than two quadrants

    T1c   Tumour involves more than two but not more than three quadrants

    T1d   Tumour involves more than three quadrants

T2   Malignant conjunctival melanoma of the non-bulbar conjunctiva involving palpebral, forniceal and/or caruncular conjunctiva

    T2a   Non-caruncular tumour involves not more than one quadrant

    T2b   Non-caruncular tumour involves more than one quadrant

    T2c   Caruncular tumour involves not more than one quadrant of conjunctiva

    T2d   Caruncular tumour involves more than one quadrant of conjunctiva

T3   Tumour with local invasion into:

    T3a   Globe

    T3b   Eyelid

    T3c   Orbit

    T3d   Sinus

T4   Tumour invades central nervous system (CNS)

Note: 1. Melanoma in situ (includes the term primary acquired melanosis) with atypia replacing greater than 75% of the normal epithelial thickness, with cytological features of epithelial cells, including abundant cytoplasm, vesicular nuclei, or prominent nucleoli, and/or presence of intraepithelial nests of atypical cells.

2. Quadrants are defined by clock hour, starting at the limbus (e.g., 6, 9, 12, 3) extending from the central cornea, to and beyond the eyelid margins. This will bisect the caruncle.

N – Regional Lymph Nodes

NX   Regional lymph nodes cannot be assessed
N0   No regional lymph node metastasis
N1   Regional lymph node metastasis

M – Distant Metastasis

M0   No distant metastasis
M1   Distant metastasis

pTNM Pathological Classification

pT – Primary Tumour

pTX   Primary tumour cannot be assessed
pT0   No evidence of primary tumour
pTis   Melanoma confined to the conjunctival epithelium (in situ)*

pT1   Melanoma of the bulbar conjunctiva
  pT1a Tumour not more than 0.5 mm in thickness with invasion of the substantia propria
  pT1b Tumour more than 0.5 mm but not more than 1.5 mm in thickness with invasion of the substantia propria
  pT1c Tumour greater than 1.5 mm in thickness with invasion of the substantia propria
pT2   Melanoma of the palpebral, forniceal, or caruncular conjunctiva

pT2a Tumour not more than 0.5 mm in thickness with invasion of the substantia propria

pT2b Tumour more than 0.5 mm but not greater than 1.5 mm in thickness with invasion of the substantia propria.

pT2c Tumour greater than 1.5 mm in thickness with invasion of the substantia propria.

pT3 Melanoma invades the eye, eyelid, nasolacrimal system, sinuses, or orbit

pT4 Melanoma invades CNS

Note: *pTis Melanoma in situ (includes the term primary acquired melanosis) with atypia replacing greater than 75% of the normal epithelial thickness, with cytological features of epithelioid cells, including abundant cytoplasm, vesicular nuclei or prominent nucleoli, and/or presence of intraepithelial nests of atypical cells.

pN – Regional Lymph Nodes

The pN categories correspond to the N categories.

pM – Distant Metastasis

For pM categories see page 15.

G Histopathological Grading

Histological grade represents the origin of the primary tumour.

GX   Origin cannot be assessed

G0   Primary acquired melanosis without cellular atypia

G1   Conjunctival nevus

G2   Primary acquired melanosis with cellular atypia (epithelial disease only)

G3   Primary acquired melanosis with epithelial cellular atypia and invasive melanoma

G4   De novo malignant melanoma

Stage Grouping

No stage grouping is at present recommended.

Summary

Malignant Melanoma of Conjunctiva			
T1	Bulbar conjunctiva	pT1	Bulbar conjunctiva
		pT1a	≤0,5mm, substantia propria
		pT1b	>0,5mm to 1,5mm, substantia propria
		pT1c	>1,5mm, substania propria
T2	Non-bulbar conjunctiva	pT2	Palpebral, forniceal, caruncular conjunctiva
		pT2a	≤0,5mm, substantia propria
		pT2b	>0,5mm to 1,5mm, subtantia propria
		pT2c	>1,5mm, substantia propria
T3	Eyelid, globe, orbit, sinuses,	pT3	Eye, eyelid, nasolacrimal system
T4	CNS	pT4	CNS

Malignant Melanoma of Uvea
(ICD-O C69.3,4)

Rules for Classification

There should be histological confirmation of the disease. The following are the procedures for assessing T, N, and M categories:

T categories	Physical examination; additional methods such as fluorescein angiography and isotope examination may enhance the accuracy of appraisal
N categories	Physical examination
M categories	Physical examination and imaging

Regional Lymph Nodes

The regional lymph nodes are the preauricular, submandibular, and cervical nodes.

Anatomical Sites

1. Iris (C69.4)
2. Ciliary body (C69.4)
3. Choroid (C69.3)

TNM Clinical Classification

T – Primary Tumour

TX   Primary tumour cannot be assessed
T0   No evidence of primary tumour

Iris*

T1   Tumour limited to iris
      T1a   Not more than 3 clock hours in size
      T1b   More than 3 clock hours in size
      T1c   With secondary glaucoma
T2   Tumour confluent with or extending into the ciliary body, choroid or both
      T2a   With secondary glaucoma
T3   Tumour confluent with or extending into the ciliary body, choroid or both, with scleral extension
      T3a   With secondary glaucoma
T4   Tumour with extrascleral extension
      T4a   Less than or equal to 5 mm in diameter
      T4b   More than 5 mm in diameter

Note: *Iris melanomas originate from, and are predominantly located in, this region of the uvea. If less than one-half of the tumour volume is located within the iris, the tumour may have originated in the ciliary body and consideration should be given to classifying it accordingly.

Ciliary Body and Choroid

Primary ciliary body and choroidal melanomas are classified according to the four tumour size categories below:

T1   Tumour size category 1
      T1a   Without ciliary body involvement and extraocular extension

Thickness (mm)	Largest basal diameter (mm)						
	<3.0	3.1–6.0	6.1–9.0	9.1–12.0	12.1–15.0	15.1–18.0	>18
>15				4	4	4	4
12.1–15.0			3	3	3	4	4
9.1–12.0		3	3	3	3	4	4
6.1–9.0	2	2	2	2	3	3	4
3.1–6.0	1	1	1	2	2	3	4
≤3.0	1	1	1	1	2	2	4

Classification for ciliary body and choroid uveal melanoma based on thickness and diameter.

T1b With ciliary body involvement

T1c Without ciliary body involvement but with extraocular extension less than or equal to 5 mm in diameter

T1d With ciliary body involvement and extraocular extension less than or equal to 5 mm in diameter

T2 Tumour size category 2

T2a Without ciliary body involvement and extraocular extension

T2b With ciliary body involvement

T2c Without ciliary body involvement but with extraocular extension less than or equal to 5 mm in diameter

T2d With ciliary body involvement and extraocular extension less than or equal to 5 mm in diameter

T3 Tumour size category 3

T3a Without ciliary body involvement and extraocular extension

T3b With ciliary body involvement

T3c Without ciliary body involvement but with extraocular extension less than or equal to 5 mm in diameter

T3d With ciliary body involvement and extraocular extension less than or equal to 5 mm in diameter

T4 Tumour size category 4

T4a Without ciliary body involvement and extraocular extension

T4b With ciliary body involvement

T4c Without ciliary body involvement but with extraocular extension less than or equal to 5 mm in diameter

T4d With ciliary body involvement and extraocular extension less than or equal to 5 mm in diameter

T4e Any tumour size category with extraocular extension more than 5 mm in diameter

*Notes: 1. In clinical practice, the largest tumour basal diameter may be estimated in optic disc diameters (dd, average: 1 dd = 1.5 mm). Tumour thickness may be estimated in diopters (average: 2.5 diopters = 1 mm). However, techniques such as ultrasonography and fundus photography are used to provide more accurate measurements. Ciliary body involvement can be evaluated by the slit-lamp, ophthalmoscopy, gonioscopy and transillumination. However, high frequency ultrasonography (ultrasound biomicroscopy) is used for more accurate assessment. Extension through the sclera is evaluated visually before and during surgery, and with ultrasonography, computed tomography or magnetic resonance imaging.

2. When histopathological measurements are recorded after fixation, tumour diameter and thickness may be underestimated because of tissue shrinkage.

N – Regional Lymph Nodes

NX   Regional lymph nodes cannot be assessed
N0   No regional lymph node metastasis
N1   Regional lymph node metastasis

M – Distant Metastasis

M0   No distant metastasis
M1   Distant metastasis

pTNM Pathological Classification

The pT and pN categories correspond to the T and N categories. For pM see page 15.

Stage Grouping

Stage I	T1a	N0	M0
Stage IIA	T1b–d, T2a	N0	M0
Stage IIB	T2b, T3a	N0	M0
Stage IIIA	T2c–d	N0	M0
	T3b–c	N0	M0
	T4a	N0	M0
Stage IIIB	T3d	N0	M0
	T4b–c	N0	M0
Stage IIIC	T4d–e	N0	M0
Stage IV	Any T	N1	M0
	Any T	Any N	M1

Summary

Uvea Malignant Melanoma

Iris Malignant Melanoma

T1	Limited to iris
T1a	≤3 clock hours
T1b	>3 clock hours
T1c	Glaucoma
T2	Into ciliary body/choroid
T2a	With glaucoma
T3	Scleral extension
T3a	With glaucoma
T4	Extraocular extension
T4a	≤5 mm
T4b	> 5 mm

Ciliary Body and Choroid Malignant Melanoma

T1	Category 1
T1a	Without extraocular extension
T1b	With microscopic extraocular extension
T1c	With gross extraocular extension
T2	Category 2
T2a	Without extraocular extension
T2b	With microscopic extraocular extension
T2c	With gross extraocular extension
T3	Category 3
T4	T3 with extraocular extension

All Sites

N1	Regional

Retinoblastoma
(ICD-O C69.2)

Rules for Classification

In bilateral cases, the eyes should be classified separately. The classification does not apply to complete spontaneous regression of the tumour. There should be histological confirmation of the disease in an enucleated eye.

The following are the procedures for assessing T, N, and M categories:

T categories	Physical examination and imaging
N categories	Physical examination
M categories	Physical examination and imaging; examination of bone marrow and cerebrospinal fluid (CSF) may enhance the accuracy of appraisal

Regional Lymph Nodes

The regional lymph nodes are the preauricular, submandibular, and cervical lymph nodes.

TNM Clinical Classification

T – Primary Tumour

TX   Primary tumour cannot be assessed
T0   No evidence of primary tumour

T1   Tumour no more than two-thirds the volume of the eye with no vitreous or subretinal seeding.

   T1a No tumour in either eye is greater than 3 mm in largest dimension or located closer than 1.5 mm to the optic nerve or fovea

   T1b At least one tumour is greater than 3 mm in largest dimension or located closer than 1.5 mm to the optic nerve or fovea. No retinal detachment or subretinal fluid beyond 5 mm from the base of the tumour

   T1c At least one tumour greater than 3 mm in largest dimension or located closer than 1.5 mm to the optic nerve or fovea, with retinal detachment or subretinal fluid beyond 5 mm from the base of the tumour

T2   Tumours no more than two-thirds the volume of the eye, or with vitreous or subretinal seeding with retinal detachment

   T2a Tumour with focal vitreous and/or subretinal seeding of fine aggregates of tumour cells, but no large clumps or 'snowballs' of tumour cells

   T2b Tumour with massive vitreous and/or subretinal seeding, defined as diffuse clumps or 'snowballs' of tumour cells

T3   Severe intraocular disease

    T3a   Tumour fills more than two-thirds of the eye

    T3b   One or more complications present, which may include tumour-associated neovascular or angle closure glaucoma, tumour extension into the anterior segment, hyphema, vitreous haemorrhage, or orbital cellulitis

T4   Extraocular tumour

    T4a   Invasion of optic nerve

    T4b   Invasion into orbit

    T4c   Intracranial extension not past chiasm

    T4d   Intracranial extension past chiasm

N – Regional Lymph Nodes

NX   Regional lymph nodes cannot be assessed

N0   No regional lymph node metastasis

N1   Regional lymph node metastasis

M – Distant Metastasis

M0   No distant metastasis

M1   Distant metastasis

TNM Pathological Classification

T – Primary Tumour

pTX   Primary tumour cannot be assessed

pT0   No evidence of primary tumour

pT1   Tumour confined to eye with no optic nerve or choroidal invasion pT2   Tumour with minimal optic nerve and/or choroidal invasion

     pT2a Tumour superficially invades optic nerve head but does not extend past lamina cribrosa *or* tumour exhibits focal choroidal invasion

     pT2b Tumour superficially invades optic nerve head but does not extend past lamina cribrosa *and* exhibits focal choroidal invasion

pT3   Tumour with significant optic nerve and/or choroidal invasion

     pT3a Tumour invades optic nerve past lamina cribrosa but not to surgical resection line *or* tumour exhibits massive choroidal invasion

     pT3b Tumour invades optic nerve past lamina cribrosa but not to surgical resection line *and* exhibits massive choroidal invasion

pT4   Tumour invades optic nerve to resection line or exhibits extraocular extension elsewhere.

     pT4a Tumour invades optic nerve to resection line but no extraocular extension identified

     pT4b Tumour invades optic nerve to resection line and extraocular extension identified

pN – Regional Lymph Nodes

pNX   Regional lymph nodes cannot be assessed

pN0   No regional lymph node involvement

pN1   Regional lymph node involvement (preauricular, cervical)

pN2   Distant lymph node involvement

pM – Metastasis

M0   No distant metastasis
pM1   Distant metastasis
pM1a Single metastasis to sites other than CNS
pM1b Multiple metastasis to sites other than CNS
pM1c CNS metastasis
pM1d Discrete mass(es) without leptomeningeal and/
      or CSF involvement
pM1e Leptomeningeal and/or Cerebral Spine Fluid
      (CSF) involvement

Stage Grouping

No stage grouping is at present recommended.

Summary

Retinoblastoma

T1	No more than 2/3 of eye volume, no vitreous/subretinal seeding	pT1	Confined to eye	
T1a	≤3 mm, ≥1.5 mm to optic nerve/fovea			
T1b	One > 3 mm or < 1.5 mm to optic nerve/fovea			
T1c	One > 3 mm or < 1.5 mm to optic nerve/fovea, retinal derachment/ subretinal fluid beyond 5 mm from tumour base			
T2	> 2/3 of eye volume with vitreous or subretinal seeding with retinal detachment	pT2	Minimal optic nerve and/or choroidal invasion	
T2a	Focal vireous and/or subretinal seeding	pT2a	Superficial invasion optic nerve	
T2b	Massive vireous and/or subretinal seeding	pT2b	Superficial invasion optic nerve, focal choroidal invasion	
T3	Severe intraocular disease	pT3	Significant invasion optic nerve and/or choroidal invasion	
T3a	> 2/3 of the eye	pT3a	Invasion of optic nerve past lamina cribrosa but not to surgical resection line *or* massive choroidal invasion	

T3b	>one complications	pT3b	Invasion of optic nerve past lamina cribrosa (not to surgical resection line, massive choroidal invasion)
T4	Extraocular tumour	pT4	Invasion of optic nerve to resection line or extraocular extension
T4a	Optic nerve	pT4a	Invasion of optic nerve to resection line, no extraocular extension
T4b	Orbit	pT4b	Invasion of optic nerve to resection Line, extraocular extension
T4c	Intracranial, not past chiasm		
T4d	Intracranial, past chiasm		
N1	Regional		
pM1	Distant metastasis		
pM1a	Single metastasis to sites other than CNS		
pM1b	Multiple metastasis to sites othe than CNS		
pM1c	CNS metastasis		
pM1d	Discrete mass(es) without leptomeningeal and/or CSF involvement		
pM1e	Leptomeningeal and/or CSF involvement		

Sarcoma of Orbit
(ICD-O C69.6)

Rules for Classification

The classification applies to sarcomas of soft tissue and bone. There should be histological confirmation of the disease and division of cases by histological type.

The following are the procedures for assessing T, N, and M categories:

T categories	Physical examination and imaging
N categories	Physical examination
M categories	Physical examination and imaging

Regional Lymph Nodes

The regional lymph nodes are the preauricular, submandibular, and cervical lymph nodes.

TNM Clinical Classification

T – Primary Tumour

TX	Primary tumour cannot be assessed
T0	No evidence of primary tumour

T1   Tumour 15 mm or less in greatest dimension

T2   Tumour more than 15 mm in greatest dimension without invasion of globe or bony wall

T3   Tumour of any size with invasion of orbital tissues and/or bony walls

T4   Tumour invades globe or periorbital structure, such as eyelids, temporal fossa, nasal cavity and paranasal sinuses, and/or CNS

N – Regional Lymph Nodes

NX   Regional lymph nodes cannot be assessed

N0   No regional lymph node metastasis

N1   Regional lymph node metastasis

M – Distant Metastasis

M0   No distant metastasis

M1   Distant metastasis

pTNM Pathological Classification

The pT and pN categories correspond to the T and N categories. For pM see page 15.

G Histopathological Grading

See definitions on page 275.

Histopathological grading of the tumour should be reported.

Stage Grouping

No stage grouping is at present recommended.

Summary

Sarcoma of Orbit	
T 1	≤15 mm
T2	>15 mm
T3	Invades orbital tissues/bony walls
T4	Invades globe or periorbital structures
N1	Regional

Carcinoma of Lacrimal Gland
(ICD-O C69.5)

Rules for Classification

There should be histological confirmation of the disease and division of cases by histological type.

The following are the procedures for assessing T, N, and M categories:

T categories	Physical examination and imaging
N categories	Physical examination
M categories	Physical examination and imaging

Regional Lymph Nodes

The regional lymph nodes are the preauricular, submandibular, and cervical lymph nodes.

TNM Clinical Classification

T – Primary Tumour

TX	Primary tumour cannot be assessed
T0	No evidence of primary tumour
T1	Tumour 2 cm or less in greatest dimension, limited to the lacrimal gland

T2   Tumour more than 2 cm but not more than 4 cm in greatest dimension, limited to the lacrimal gland

T3   Tumour more than 4 cm or with extraglandular extension into orbital soft tissue, including optic nerve or globe

T4   Tumour invades periosteum or orbital bone or adjacent structures

      T4a   Tumour invades periosteum

      T4b   Tumour invades orbital bone

      T4c   Tumour invades adjacent structures (brain, sinus, pterygoid fossa, temporal fossa)

N – Regional Lymph Nodes

NX   Regional lymph nodes cannot be assessed

N0   No regional lymph node metastasis

N1   Regional lymph node metastasis

M – Distant Metastasis

M0   No distant metastasis

M1   Distant metastasis

pTNM Pathological Classification

The pT and pN categories correspond to the T and N categories. For pM see page 15.

G Histopathological Grading

GX   Grade of differentiation cannot be assessed

G1   Well differentiated

G2   Moderately differentiated; includes adenoid cystic carcinoma without basaloid (solid) pattern

G3   Poorly differentiated; includes adenoid cystic carcinoma with basaloid (solid) pattern

G4   Undifferentiated

Stage Grouping

No stage grouping is at present recommended.

Summary

Lacrimal Gland Carcinoma	
T1	≤2 cm, limited to gland
T2	>2.0 cm to 4 cm, limited to gland
T3	>4 cm, extraglandular extension into orbital soft tissue including optic nerve or globe
T4	Periosteum, orbital bone, adjacent structures
T4a	Periosteum
T4b	Orbit bone
T4c	Adjacent structures
N1	Regional

HODGKIN LYMPHOMA

Introductory Notes

At the present time it is not considered practical to propose a TNM classification for Hodgkin lymphoma.

Following the development of the Ann Arbor classification for Hodgkin lymphoma in 1971, the significance of two important observations with major impact on staging has been appreciated. First, extra-lymphatic disease, if localized and related to adjacent lymph node disease, does not adversely affect the survival of patients. Second, laparotomy with splenectomy has been introduced as a method of obtaining more information on the extent of the disease within the abdomen.

A stage classification based on information from histopathological examination of the spleen and lymph nodes obtained at laparotomy cannot be compared with another without such exploration. Therefore, two systems of classification are presented, a clinical (cS) and a pathological (pS).

Clinical Staging (cS)

Clinical stage describes the anatomic extent of Hodgkin lymphoma and forms the basis for treatment decision. It is determined by history, clinical examination, imaging, and blood analysis. Bone marrow biopsy is indicated in selected cases and must be taken from a clinically or radiologically or non-involved area of bone.

Liver Involvement

Clinical evidence of liver involvement must include either enlargement of the liver and at least an abnormal serum alkaline phosphatase level and two different liver function test abnormalities, or an abnormal liver demonstrated by imaging and one abnormal liver function test.

Spleen Involvement

Clinical evidence of spleen involvement is accepted if there is palpable enlargement of the spleen confirmed by imaging.

Lymphatic and Extralymphatic Disease

The lymphatic structures are as follows:

- Lymph nodes
- Waldeyer ring
- Spleen
- Appendix
- Thymus
- Peyer patches

The lymph nodes are grouped into regions and one or more (2, 3, etc.) may be involved. The spleen is designated S and extralymphatic organs or sites E.

Lung Involvement

Lung involvement limited to one lobe, or perihilar extension associated with ipsilateral lymphadenopathy, or unilateral pleural effusion with or without lung involvement but with hilar lymphadenopathy is considered as *localized* extralymphatic disease.

Liver Involvement

Liver involvement is always considered as *diffuse* extralymphatic disease.

Pathological Staging (pS)

Pathological stage follows clinical stage with clinical information supplemented by the information obtained from staging laparotomy and splenectomy. Since the current approach to treatment almost always includes systemic treatment, staging laparotomy is no longer performed and pathological staging is usually not available.

Histopathological Information

This is classified by symbols indicating the tissue sampled. The following notation is common to the distant metastases (or M1 categories) of all regions classified by the TNM system. However, in order to conform with the Ann Arbor classification, the initial letters used in that system are also given.

Pulmonary	PUL or L	Bone marrow	MAR or M
Osseous	OSS or O	Pleura	PLE or P
Hepatic	HEP or H	Peritoneum	PER
Brain	BRA	Adrenals	ADR
Lymph nodes	LYM or N	Skin	SKI or D
Others	OTH		

Clinical Stages (cS)

Stage I

Involvement of a single lymph node region (I), or localized involvement of a single extralymphatic organ or site (I_E)

Stage II

Involvement of two or more lymph node regions on the same side of the diaphragm (II), or localized involvement of a single extralymphatic organ or site and its regional lymph node(s) with or without involvement of other lymph node regions on the same side of the diaphragm (II_E)

Note: The number of lymph node regions involved may be indicated by a subscript (e.g., II_4, page 304.)

Stage III

Involvement of lymph node regions on both sides of the diaphragm (III), which may also be accompanied by localized involvement of an associated extralymphatic organ or site III_E, or by involvement of the spleen (III_S), or both III_{E+S}.

Stage IV

Disseminated (multifocal) involvement of one or more extralymphatic organs, with or without associated lymph node involvement; or isolated extralymphatic organ involvement with distant (non-regional) nodal involvement.

Note: The site of Stage IV disease is identified further by specifying sites according to the notations listed above.

A and B Classification (Symptoms)

Each stage should be divided into A and B according to the absence or presence of defined general symptoms. These are:

1. Unexplained weight loss of more than 10% of the usual body weight in the 6 months prior to first attendance
2. Unexplained fever with temperature above 38°C
3. Night sweats

Note: Pruritus alone does not qualify for B classification nor does a short, febrile illness associated with a known infection.

Pathological Stages (pS)

The definitions of the four stages follow the same criteria as the clinical stages but with the additional information obtained following laparotomy. Splenectomy, liver biopsy, lymph node biopsy, and marrow biopsy are mandatory for the establishment of pathological stages.

Summary

Stage	Hodgkin Lymphoma	Substage
Stage I	Single node region	
	Localized single extra-lymphatic organ/site	I_E
Stage II	Two or more node regions, same side of diaphragm	II_E
	Localized single extra-lymphatic organ/ site with its regional nodes, $\pm$ other node regions same side of diaphragm	
Stage III	Node regions both sides of diaphragm	III_E
	+ localized single extra-lymphatic organ/site	
	Spleen	III_S
	Both	III_{E+S}
Stage IV	Diffuse or multifocal involvement of extra-lymphatic organ(s) $\pm$ regional nodes; isolated extralymphatic organ and non-regional nodes	
All stages divided	Without weight loss/ fever/sweats	A
	With weight loss/ fever/sweats	B

NON-HODGKIN LYMPHOMAS

The staging classification for non-Hodgkin lymphomas is the same as for Hodgkin lymphomas (see page 304).